Obstetric Surgery • Egbert H. Gran Wallace Jarman

Publisher's Note

The book descriptions we ask booksellers to display prominently warn that this is an historic book with numerous typos or missing text; it is not indexed or illustrated.

The book was created using optical character recognition software. The software is 99 percent accurate if the book is in good condition. However, we do understand that even one percent can be an annoying number of typos! And sometimes all or part of a page may be missing from our copy of the book. Or the paper may be so discolored from age that it is difficult to read. We apologize and gratefully acknowledge Google's assistance.

After we re-typeset and design a book, the page numbers change so the old index and table of contents no longer work. Therefore, we often remove them; otherwise, please ignore them.

Our books sell so few copies that you would have to pay hundreds of dollars to cover the cost of our proof reading and fixing the typos, missing text and index. Instead we let most customers download a free copy of the original typo-free scanned book. Simply enter the barcode number from the back cover of the paperback in the Free Book form at www.RareBooksClub.com. You may also qualify for a free trial membership in our book club to download up to four books for free. Simply enter the barcode number from the back cover onto the membership form on our home page. The book club entitles you to select from more than a million books at no additional charge. Simply enter the title or subject onto the search form to find the books.

If you have any questions, could you please be so kind as to consult our Frequently Asked Questions page at www.RareBooksClub.com/faqs.cfm? You are also welcome to contact us there.

General Books LLC™, Memphis, USA, 2012.

EGBERT H. GRANDIN, M.D.,
Obstetric Schoeon To The N-ew Yorr Maternity Hospital; GtnJtcolocist To The
French Hospital, Etc.;
AND
GEORGE W. JARMAN, M.D.,
Obstetric Surgeon To The New Yorr Maternitt Hospital; Gtn.«cologist To The
Cancer Hospital, Etc.

With Eighty-Five Illustrations in the Text and Fifteen Photographic Plates.
i
PREFACE.

The key-note of this volume is *election* in obstetric surgery.

The results which are daily secured in general surgery through resort to timely operation are obtainable in obstetrics if the same principle be held in view.

This volume, further, being written from a teaching basis, is necessarily imbued with the personality of the authors, and is, therefore, not burdened with literature references and statistical data. The latter have alone been introduced, when necessary, in order to assist in the elucidation of some disputed point.

The illustrations have been prepared and selected with the special end in view of teaching graphically. The works of Barnes, Charpentier, Lusk, Cazeaux, and Oscar Schaeffer, in particular, have furnished many of the wood-cuts, and the authors hereby express their obligation. The photographic plates have been prepared from nature under the personal supervision of the authors.

On the basis of honest desire to promote progress in obstetrics, this volume is offered to the medical profession.

September, 185i.
CONTENTS.
INTRODUCTION.
PAGE
Obstetric Asepsis And Antisepsis, I

Obstetric Dystocia And Its Determination, 9
CHAPTER II.
Artificial Abortion And The Induction Of Premature Labor,. 34
CHAPTER III.
The Forceps, 72
CHAPTER IV.
YER8ION, 93
CHAPTER V.
Symphysiotomy 120
CHAPTER VI.
The Cesarean Section, 132
CHAPTER VII.
Embryotomy.. 146
CHAPTER VIII.
The Surgery Of The Puerperium 163
CHAPTER IX.
Ectopic (jestation, 193
Index 203

LIST OF ILLUSTRATIONS.
no. PAGE 1. Normal female pelvis 9 2. Beaudeloeque's pelvimeter, 10 3. Martin's pelvimeter, 10 4. Schultze's pelvimeter, 11 5. Collyer's poeket pelvimeter, 11 6. Justo-major pelvis 18 7. Generally equally contracted pelvis (justo-minor), 19 8. Flat iion-rachitic pelvis, 20 9. Flat rachitic pelvis (mild grade), 21 10. Flat rachitic pelvis (high grade), 22 11. Generally contracted Hat rachitic pelvis, 23 12. Roberts's pelvis. The transversely contracted pelvis, 24 13. The kyphotic pelvis, showing narrowing in the transverse diameter and length ening In the conjugate, 25 14. Non-rachitic scoliotic skeleton, 26 15. Rachitic scoliotic skeleton, 26 16. Spondylolisthetic pelvis 27 17. The osteomalacic pelvis 29 18. Obliquely distorted pelvis of Naegele 30 19. Osteosarcoma of the pelvis, 32 20. Steel-branched dilator, 41 21. Uterine curette, 41 22. Ovum forceps, 42 23. Glass Irrigating tube, 42 24. Fritsch-Bozeman catheter, 42 25. Edebohl's speculum, 43 26. Cervical tenaculum, 43 27. Intrauterine dressing forceps, 45 28. Barnes's bags, 66 29. McLean's bag, 66

30. Marx's incubator (closed), 70 31. Marx's Incubator (open), 71 32. Elliott forceps, 72 33. Hunter forceps, 73 34. Lusk-Tarnier forceps 73 35. Jewett's axis-traction forceps 74 30. Showing Reynolds's traction rods in position, 75 37. Introduction of the left blade of the forceps, 79 38. The left blade introduced; the right blade (in outline) ready to be introduced,. 80 39. The forceps adjusted and ready to be locked, 81 40. Showing the direction of the line of traction,.83 41. Showing direction of traction in face presentation, 86 42. Tarnler forceps applied to the thighs, 88 43. Incision of the cervix, 89 44. Application of medium forceps, 90 viii LIST OF ILLUSTRATIONS.

Fig. PAGE 45. First stage of bipolar version 102 46. Grasping the knee, 103 47. Representing first act of extraction, 104 48. Version in head presentation, 106 49. Completing the version, 107 50. Impacted shoulder, 108 51. Introduction of the left hand to bring down the posterior (left) leg,... 109 52. Showing direction of traction, 110 53. Method of releasing the cord, Ill 54. Disengagement of the posterior (right) arm 112 55. Showing direction of traction, 113 56. The child is lifted over the perineum and the occiput passes from under the sym physis,. .. 114 57. Chin arrested at symphysis 115 58. Forceps applied to after-coming head, 116 59. The bulging of peritoneum and of bladder into the opening at the joint,.. 128 60. Galblati-Harris Knife. (Harris's modification), 124 61. Showing deep suture passed, the loops not cut, 138 02. The same, the loops cut, 138 63. Suture of uterine wound, 139 64. Braun's trephine, 148 65. Blot's perforator, 148 66. Martin's trephine, 149 67. Scissors-perforator, 149 68. Braun's cranioclast 149 69. Effect of the cranioclast on the foetal skull, 151 70. Lusk's cephalotribe, 154 71. Tarnier's basioti ibe, 1.54 72. Bono-forceps, 157 73. Crochet and blunt hook, 157 74. Braun's hook or decollator, 158 75. Delivery of trunk after section of head, 159 76. Locked twins 160 77. Sutures inserted on one side of a lacerated cervix, 166 78. Insertion of sutures. (After Hegar.), 171 79. Laceration through the sphincter. Sphincter sutures in place,.... 172 80. Repair of a vesico-vaginal fistula, 174 81. Simon's specula, 175 82. Transverse rupture of the uterus, 179 83. Cleveland's ligature-carrier, 197 84. Emergency Trendelenburg posture, 198 LIST OF FULL-PAGE PLATES.

PAGE
Plate I.—Measurement of distance between the spines,.... 12

Plate II.—Fig. 1. Measurement of Beaudelocque diameter. Fig. 2. Measurement of Beaudelocque diameter in ease of pendulous abdomen, 12

Plate III.—Fig. 1. Determination of the diagonal conjugate. Fig. 2. Depression of the uterus so as to determine adaptability of presenting part to the pelvic brim, 14

Plate IV.—Introduction of the left blade of the forceps,... 79

Plate V.—Fig. 1. Towel applied to handle of Hunter's forceps. Fig. 2. Bilateral incision of the perineum (episiotoiuy),.... 82

Plate VI.—Showing method of grasping the foot, 109

Plate VII.—Extracting the posterior leg, 109

Plate VIII.—Extracting the posterior arm, 112

Plate IX.—Head impacted at the outlet. Admitting air that the child may breathe, 115

Plate X.—The child is lifted over the perineum and the occiput passes from under the symphysis. An assistant makes suprapubic pressure, 115

Plate XI.—Traction while the head is in the transverse diameter of the pelvis, 116

Plate "II.—Application of the forceps to the after-coming head,.. 116

Platf XIII.—Method of grasping the child's body in performing internal rotation 118

Plate XIV.Fig. 1. Trephining the before-coming head. Fig. 2. Perforation of the after-coming head, 150

Plate XV.—Insertion of Braun's decollator,...... 158

Obstetric Surgery. INTRODUCTION.
OBSTETRIC ASEPSIS AND ANTISEPSIS.

It is only within the last decade that obstetric surgery has progressed toward the scientific eminence to which it may justly lay claim to-day. Before the advent of the era of antisepsis and asepsis, before the fear of handling the uterus had been swept away, the forceps and version were the only operations which came within the ken of the average practitioner, and the results from resort to these were anything than matters to be proud of. So-called childbed fever was virulent not alone after spontaneous labor at term, but also after resort to any and all obstetric operations.

To-day the scene has radically changed. Septica;mia after labor is justly considered as due, in almost every instance, to faulty asepsis; gradually bettering attempts are being made to educate the student with a practical knowledge of the entire range of obstetric surgery, and extra stress is being laid, as it should be, on the absolute necessity of studying the pelvis of the pregnant woman before the advent of labor, so as to be in a position to take advantage of that operative procedure, where any is indicated, which is best not alone for the woman, but which also takes into account the welfare of the child. Whilst, then, more accurate educational methods enter as factors in the science of obstetrics as practiced to-day, the fundamental reason why mortality rate has been lowered is the recognition of the culpability of the man who neglects the laws of cleanliness (asepsis and antisepsis) throughout the conduct of labor and during the puerperal state. Lack of cleanliness (asepsis and antisepsis) will ruin the most expert technique, and, therefore, a thorough grounding in the fundamental laws of cleanliness as applied to obstetric work is essential to the undertaking of any of the surgery of the art.

Antisepsis is simply the means of certifying to asepsis (cleanliness). The whole question has been needlessly complicated by the introduction of scores of chemical agents which possess, to a greater or less degree, the power of rendering inert the micro-organisms which exist in, or may be conveyed to, the human body. It is possible to secure asepsis without resorting to antisepsis, but, in order to surround surgery with every possible safeguard, these chemical agents must be looked upon as absolutely essential. The point to be remembered in obstetric surgery is that too free indulgence in antisepsis may do harm even whilst it aims at good. The nature of many of the antiseptic agents on which we must needs rely is poisonous to the human body. Therefore the corollary must be borne in mind that overzealousness in matters of antisepsis may injure and kill, even as lack of asepsis may be followed by similar effects. Obstetric asepsis is secured through attention to (a) the person of the accoucheur, the nurse, and assistants; *(b)* the lying-in woman; (c) the instruments and accessories.

(«) Asepsis Of The Accoucheur And Attendants.

It being absolutely proven that septicaemia is heterogenetic, —that is to say, does not originate within the body,—it is the bounden duty of all who come in direct contact with the lying-in woman to keep themselves not alone clean, but also free from those acute infectious elements which, through inoculation, breed sepsis. The ideal obstetrician, like the ideal surgeon, should avoid seeing patients suffering from certain of the acute infectious diseases, such as scarlet fever and diphtheria; and, except in absolute emergency, should have nothing to do with post mortem examinations. These rules of conduct should be absolute with the expert obstetrician, who, from recognized standing, is liable at any time to be called upon to give advice in the minor emergencies of labor or to act as chief in major operative obstetrics. Barring spontaneous or operative traumatic lesions, the risk the lying-in woman runs is septic infection at the hands of her immediate attendants. The general practitioner of necessity must perform obstetric work even whilst his routine duty calls for attendance on scarlet fever, for instance. The greater, therefore, the precautions he should take to bathe thoroughly, to change his garments, to wash his hair and beard, to asepticize his hands before going from such diseased states to a woman who is about to perform a physiological act. In the event of his time being occupied to a great degree with attention to patients sick from any of the acute infectious diseases, so that he finds it difficult to take the simple and yet most essential precautions mentioned above, then it is wise, to say no more, for the time being to refuse to attend labor cases, else, as has too frequently happened, one puerpera after another will be diseased, if not killed. The man who makes postmortems frequently is a death-dealing obstetrician, and the careless general practitioner may become such. It has been well said, and cannot be emphasized too strongly, that puerperal sepsis means faulty technique,—that is to say, one or more of the attendants are to blame. There is no shifting the responsibility on nature.

Such general measures as have been noted apply with even greater force to the nurse. She will come more frequently in contact with the woman, and, if careless, is even more likely to septicize. If ignorant, as outside of large centres she is apt to be, she may even now, in this aseptic age, fill grave-yards as she did in the past. It becomes, therefore, the duty of the physician to investigate the previous occupation and whereabouts of the nurse his patient has engaged, and to insist on her practicing the most rigorous antisepsis as regards her clothing and person. Asepsis is not sufficient for the average nurse; she must be provided with antiseptics in order to cause her to approximate cleanliness. It goes without saying that she should never be allowed to attend the lying-in woman if she has been, within at least a week, in attendance on one of the acute infectious diseases. The rigid rules about to be noted as applicable to the care of the obstetric hands are to be enforced with her even as they must be with the physician.

In the lying-in room the physician should remove his coat and roll up his shirt-sleeves above the elbow. Since, aside from instruments, the hands are most likely to septicize the woman from direct contact, great care must be exercised to render them aseptic. If the physician has recently been in contact with any infectious material, thorough washing in soap and water and scrubbing in bichloride solution will not suffice to render these hands aseptic. Under such conditions the following method must be resorted to: The hands and arms are scrubbed for at least ten minutes in hot soap and water, the latter being frequently changed. Especial attention must be paid to the fingernails, under which the infectious elements are most prone to lodge. The hands and the arms are next covered with a hot saturated solution of permanganate of potash, and are then immersed in a hot saturated solution of oxalic acid until the stain of the permanganate has entirely disappeared. The oxalic acid is next removed by soaking the hands in hot sterilized water.

If the physician be at all suspicious about the nurse, she should be compelled to resort to the same process under his direct supervision. It has been proven by culture experiments that this method of treating the hands renders them absolutely free from micro-organisms.

Under ordinary conditions, where the physician is sure of his freedom from infectious material, this elaborate process is not necessary. It will suffice to scrub the hands in hot soap and water, and next to immerse them in a 1 to 1000 solution of bichloride of mercury. They are then washed in alcohol. After this sterilization of the hands the physician must avoid touching anything which has not been similarly sterilized.

Before proceeding to the performance of any obstetric manipulation, the physician should cover his clothing with a clean sheet, which may be found in even the households of the most indigent.

(6) Asepsis Of The Lying-in Woman.

Thorough asepsis of the genital tract of the woman is most essential, and, at the same time, most difficult to secure. These organs must be rendered surgically clean, and yet the means resorted to must be such as will not injure the protecting coat of epithelium. It is very questionable if douching of the genitals is sufficient for asepsis. The antiseptic agents thus employed at best only come in contact with the superficies. The vagina, in particular, is rendered aseptic with difficulty. It is in the depths of the rugosities that the micro-organisms lodge. Before undertaking any surgical manipulation the following means should be resorted to: The external genitals are to be scrubbed with hot soap and water, and next washed with a solution of bichloride (1 to 1000). If the required manipulations are in the vagina, a new tooth-brush should be inserted into the canal, and this should also be scrubbed with soap and water. It is next to be scrubbed with a solution of bichloride of mercury (1 to 1000).

In the event of the proposed operation being a symphysiotomy or a Caesarean section, the pubes must be shaved, the skin thoroughly washed with soap and water, then washed with bichloride solution (1 to 1000), and finally with alcohol or with ether. After any manipulation in the uterus, in order to certify to perfect post-operative technique, the entire genital tract should be douched with bichloride solution (1 to 5000). There is risk of poisoning if stronger solutions than this are used in the uterus.

(c) Asepsis Of Instruments And Accessories.

The elaborate processes which are in use in hospitals obviously cannot be resorted to in private practice. Just as thorough asepsis, however, as regards instruments, may be secured if these instruments have been carefully cleansed by the physician before they are taken to the woman's house. Instruments which have been scrubbed with soap and water, and next boiled for ten minutes in a 1-per-cent. solution of carbonate of soda (the common washing-soda), may be deemed aseptic. This asepticism, however, is destroyed if they are then placed in the average obstetric bag, which contains bottles and cotton, and, from old age, micro-organisms of every possible genus.

The sterilized instruments must be wrapped in a sterilized napkin or towel before they are placed in the bag, and immediately before use must be again washed in hot soap-suds and next boiled in the 1-per-cent. soda solution. In every household the washing-soda will be found, as well as the pot in which to boil them. The instruments may be used directly from this soda solution or else may be first transferred, with aseptic hands, into a 5-per-cent. solution of creolin,—a solution which is an efficient antiseptic and yet will not injure the instruments as does bichloride. This creolin further answers the purpose of an emollient. If there is one thing more dangerous to the patient than another, it is the vasclin which it is customary to use as an emollient. The vaselin-pot should, once and for all, be banished from the lying-in chamber. If newly opened it may not contain micro-organisms, but when it has been repeatedly exposed to the air, and possibly has been used scores of times, it will be found a veritable culture-medium for bacteria. Creolin will answer as a lubricant for the finger and for the instruments, and this should be the only lubricant allowed in the lying-in room, unless the physician prefers to use sterilized oil.

As far as is possible the physician should avoid using rubber instruments. It is difficult to render them sterile. The stronger antiseptics will ruin them, the weaker will not asepticize them. Prolonged boiling may sterilize them, but often at the expense of their integrity and, therefore, of their utility. Glass catheters and glass irrigating-tubes should be selected. These may be boiled, and thus be rendered safe to use. The metal catheter, which the average nurse will produce with pride, should be taken from her and returned only when she leaves the case, and then with the injunction to either throw it away or to lock it up and to forget it. Many a case of puerperal cystitis has been traced to the use of this relic of pre-aseptic days.

During the performance of an obstetric operation sponges should not be used. This is another article which should have no foothold in the modern lying-in room. Sterilized towels and sterilized gauze or absorbent cotton should take the place of the sponge. In every household, no matter how humble, there is an oven, and in this towels and gauze may be baked. If the oven is lacking, there always exists a means for boiling them.

For purposes of irrigation boiled water should be used. To this creolin may be added to make a 2-per-cent. solution, except where it is essential to see the irrigated portion, and then, since the milk-white creolin solution will obscure vision, bichloride solution (1 to 5000) must be substituted.

Ligature and suture material must be absolutely sterile. In view of the difficulty of obtaining sterile catgut it is wise never to use it. The ideal suture is silk-worm gut. If this be boiled for ten minutes in creolin—5-pcr-cent. solution—it is rendered aseptic, and is further rendered pliable. Obstetric surgery being often emergency surgery, the operator has not the time to prepare beforehand his catgut and silk so as to feel certain about them. Further, since the major portion of obstetric work falls to the lot of the busy general practitioner, his precedent preparations must be as simple as is consistent with absolute asepticism.

If these simple rules for securing asepsis of the lying-in woman and her surroundings are followed, the morbidity rate and mortality rate in private practice will approximate those which are secured to-day in maternity hospitals, where the mortality rate has been reduced to a fractional percentage, and where morbidity from sepsis is practically abolished. We have endeavored to emphasize our belief, and this is the current belief, that the lying-in woman is septicized solely through personal contact. By this we mean that the atmosphere is not a factor, and that the infectious material does not originate in the body of the woman. The sole exception to this latter statement is where, during the progress of labor or during obstetric manipulation, a pyosalpinx, for instance, ruptures. Such an event may lead to septic infection of the woman, but then the sepsis cannot be properly considered an obstetric epi-phenomenon.

Aseptic and *elective* obstetrics rob labor of its terrors and the puerperal state of well-nigh its sole risk.

CHAPTER I. OBSTETRIC DYSTOCIA AND ITS DETERMINATION.

A Scientific knowledge of the configuration of the female pelvis and of the methods of estimating its capacity is an essential prelude to the practice of midwifery. The surgical side of the art, in particular, rests its results on accurate pelvimetry. The fate of the woman and of the foetus is intimately linked with the expertness of the physician in determining, before or at the time of labor, the probable capacity of the pelvis in its relation to the estimated size of the foetus. A consideration, therefore, of the surgical means at our disposal for assisting labor or for facing its emergencies, must be preceded by a careful study of the pelvis, normal and abnormal.

Furthermore, the pelvis is not the only element in the problem which is to be solved. An approximate idea of the size of the foetus which is to pass through the birth-canal is also to be secured. It is essential, therefore, to precede the surgery of parturition by a description in brief of the anatomy of the obstetric pelvis and of the general physical features of the foetus.

The pelvis is formed by the union of the ossa innominata with the sacrum. The sacrum is connected with the vertebral column above and with the coccyx below. The resulting canal is larger above than below, and is flattened to a degree from in front backward. The superior, wider portion constitutes the greater pelvis, the inferior and narrower portion the lesser pelvis. The pelvis is further subdivided into a number of straits, the entrance into the canal receiving the name of superior strait, the median portion constituting the middle strait, the exit from the canal the inferior strait. It is the determination of the measurements in various directions of these three portions which is termed pelvimetry, and the resultants constitute the diameters of the pelvis. The diameters of the pelvis are to be obtained both externally and internally, and the former stand in a certain relation to the latter.

Instruments For The Determination Of The Pelvic Diameters.

The best-known pelvimeter is that devised by Beaudelocque. In view of the fact, however, that the instrument should be portable, the Martin pelvimeter will be found preferable. It should ever be remembered that the pelvimeter is as indispensable to the obstetrician as is the microscope to the physiologist, and, therefore, that it should be associated with pregnancy in his mind as the forceps is with labor. (Figs. 2, 3, 4, and 5.)

External Diameters Of Pelvis.

The following external diameters are of chief obstetric significance: The distance between the anterior superior spines of the ilium, that between the crests of the ilium, that between the trochanters, that between the spinous process of the last lumbar vertebra and the centre of the anterior surface of the pubic bones (the diameter of Beaudeloeque). These are the essential measurements which are to be obtained by means of the pelvimeter. The objection which has, over and over again, been made to this instrument, that the patient will object to the exposure which it entails, will not hold, for the reason that there need be none, as the patient is covered by a sheet; and, instead of there being objection made, the patient will have a higher opinion of the physician who evidently is taking every requisite precaution for her future safety. It cannot be emphasized too strongly that the physician is to-day not guiltless who, whenever it may be, does not practice pelvimetry. (See Plates I and II.)

In using this or any similar instrument the utmost care must be exercised to adapt the points of the blades accurately to the soft parts (as is purposely shown in the plates), and, in instances where it is of considerable importance to determine with great accuracy the exact measurements, it is advisable that these should be taken by two persons independently. These external measurements, of course, give us purely a relative idea of the internal, but, occasionally, a slight diminution beyond the normal in one or another diameter, may turn the scale in favor of one over another obstetric operation.

The following external measurements may be taken as normal in the average case, although it should ever be remembered that the estimated capacity of a given pelvis depends on the estimated size of the foetus which must pass through it:—

Distance between the spines,.. 10 to 10£ inches.

Distance between the crests,.. 10 to 11 inches.

Distance between the trochanters,. 12 to 12 inches.

Diameter of Beaudeloeque,.... 8 inches.

The must important of these external diameters is that of Beaudeloeque. By means of this external conjugate we are enabled to approximate the true conjugate,—that is to say, the diameter of the pelvic inlet,—the distance from the

Fig. 2.—Measurement of Beaudelocque Diameter in Case of Pendulous Abdomen.

upper margin of the pubic symphysis to the promontory of the sacrum. In general it may be stated that a mean deduction of three inches from the measurement of the external conjugate will give us that of the true conjugate. As regards the other external diameters, suffice it to say that diminution below the foregoing measurements, which represent a mean from a large number of pelves examined, should always be a source of thought and solicitude to the physician. This matter will be amply considered under the heading of the various operations.

Internal Diameters Of Pelvis.

Many instruments have been devised for determining the internal diameters. The finger and, if need be, the hand of the physician best subserve the purpose. Obviously, the hand can only be used under anaesthesia; but in every instance where the determination of the internal diameters is of moment in the selection of one operative procedure over another, in view of the almost absolute safety of anaesthesia, this should be resorted to. In the vast majority of cases, however, digital pelvimetry yields us sufficiently exact information in regard to the capacity of the pelvis. This should be practiced as a routine measure in every case. We may thus determine the diagonal conjugate, and, this having been obtained, the true conjugate is readily ascertained by deducting the estimated depth of the pubic symphysis. The transverse and oblique diameters may also be thus approximately measured. To perform digital pelvimetry the patient should occupy the dorsal position, with the nates on the very edge of the bed or couch. The index and the middle finger of the right hand are introduced into the vagina, the perineum being depressed as much as possible. The aim of the fingers is to reach the junction of the sacrum with the last lumbar vertebra, for it is the distance from this point to the lower margin of the symphysis pubis which yields the diagonal conjugate. If the sacral promontory cannot be reached, the inference is safe that the pelvis is normal as regards its antero-posterior diameter. If the promontory can be reached, then the wrist is carried upward until the edge of the index finger rests against the pubic symphysis. The index of the other hand notes this subpubic point, the fingers are withdrawn, and, by means of a tape-measure or the pelvimeter, the distance from the end of the middle finger to the noted point on the edge of the index is measured. This measurement is the sacro-subpubic or the diagonal conjugate diameter. (Plate III, Fig. 1.)

According to the estimated depth and obliquity of the symphysis in a given case, it is necessary to deduct from one-fourth to one-half an inch from this measurement, in order to obtain the dimension of the sacro-suprapubic or true conjugate of the pelvis.

In taking the above measurement it should be remembered that occasionally the first sacral vertebra projects over the second, forming a false promontory. To avoid mistaking this for the true sacral promontory, it is only necessary to depress the perineum or to carry the fingers as high upward as possible. Then, in the event of the existence of a false promontory, the true will be found above it.

The transverse and the oblique diameters of the pelvis cannot be measured with the same exactitude as the conjugate. As a general rule, it may be stated that, when the promontory cannot be reached in a symmetrical pelvis, labor at term is possible with a foetus of average size. If there be a suspicion, however, of a deviation from the normal in the pelvis, then the welfare of the woman and the fœtus calls for anaesthesia, in order that the entire hand may be inserted into the vagina, so that the capacity of the pelvis may be determined. This point cannot be emphasized too strongly. The scientific determination of the operative procedure to be elected in the presence of an abnormal pelvis depends on pelvimetry as accurate as possible. The instruments which from time to time have been devised for the purpose of internal pelvimetry cannot take the

F.g. 2.—DcprtSMOn of the Uterus so as to Determine Adaptability of P esentin Part to the Pelvic B r. m

Fig-2.—Depression of the Uterus so as to Determine Adaptability of Presenting Part to the Pelvic Brim.

place of the finger and hand; further, outside of maternity hospitals these instruments will rarely be at the disposal of the practitioner. Usually, fortunately, the careful measurement of the external diameters of the pelvis and the accurate estimation of the true conjugate will give a sufficient estimate of the capacity of the pelvis. Where the estimate thus obtained falls below the normal, we repeat, manual pelvimetry under anaesthesia is called for. Further, in the presence of a contracted pelvis, we thus not alone note the capacity of and shape of the pelvis, but we also—and this is of equal importance—may form an approximate idea of the size of the foetal presenting part. (Plate III, Fig. 2.) Whilst the hand is in the pelvis the uterus may be depressed, and the facility with which the presenting part is likely to engage within the pelvic inlet may be noted. Far too little stress is laid on the relation which the fœtus bears to the canal through which it must pass into the world. A given pelvis may be large enough, although diminished in all its diameters, for a foetus below the average size, and the reverse is equally true. Could we solve as approximately the size of the foetus as we can the capacity of the pelvis, the surgical side of obstetrics would be much simplified. As yet, however, we may only form an imperfect and relative idea of the ease with which the foetal presenting part will enter the pelvic canal. In general, however, if a foetus can engage at the pelvic inlet the chances are that it can engage at the outlet, unless, indeed, the alteration in shape of this outlet is marked enough to be determined even by digital pelvimetry.

Aside from the conjugate, the internal diameters of the pelvis which the practitioner should estimate in the average case are as follow, with the dimensions necessary for the birth of the average foetus:—

Diameters. Brim. Cavity. Outlet.
Transverse,. 5 in. 5 to 5£ in. 4f in.
Oblique,... 4£ to 5 in. 5 to b in. 4f in.
Conjugate,. 4£ to 4£ in. 4 in. 5 in.

It will be noted from these figures that in the normal pelvis the transverse diameter is widest at the brim and narrowest at the outlet; the oblique is widest in the cavity and narrowest at the outlet; the antero-posterior is widest at the outlet and narrowest at the brim. Therefore, a foetus of average size, engaging normally at the brim, can pass without assistance through the cavity and emerge at the outlet, if the estimate of the pelvic capacity do not fall below these figures. Where the obtained measurements are below these figures, we are in face of an abnormal pelvis, and the degree of abnormality in relation to the estimated size of the foetus must be carefully weighed before we are in a position to determine the measures, if any, which are requisite for the safe conduct of the labor.

A further measurement to be taken is the circumference. This is chiefly of importance in determining asymmetry of the pelvis. The circumference may be secured by means of a tapemeasure. Failing this the pelvimeter may be utilized by measuring each lateral half separately. This latter method will best enable us to secure knowledge in reference to pelvic asymmetry.

Before entering into a consideration of deviation of the pelvis from the normal, it is essential to recall briefly the average dimensions of the foetus at term, for, as already stated, the practitioner must take into account in his estimate not alone the probable capacity of the given pelvis, but also the probable size of the body which must pass through this pelvis.

The weight of the average foetus at term varies from 6½ to pounds, and the length is about 20 inches. The chief diameters of the foetal head, with their measurements, are:—

Occipitofrontal, 4 inches.
Occipitomental,......-b inches.
Cervico-bregmatic, 3J inches.
Frontomental,........ 3£ inches.
Suboccipito-bregmatic, 3£ inches.
Biparietal, 3J inches.

It should ever be remembered that during the course of labor some of these diameters, owing chiefly to the presence of the fontanelles, are capable of diminution, always, however, at the expense of others. In the course of a normal labor the molding of the foetal head as it descends flexes and rotates in the pelvis, results in diminution of those diameters which adapt themselves to the most favorable diameters of the pelvis, and the corollary is that in case of abnormal pelvis the aim of the attendant should be to guide the longest diameters of the fœtal head into the longest diameters of the pelvic canal. Such an aim presupposes accurate knowledge of pelvic configuration, and hence a further reason for accurate pelvimetry in every case. The problem before the physician is rarely a simple one, and as we pass from a consideration of the normal pelvis to that of the abnormal pelvis this problem becomes all the more complex.

General Considerations Of Abnormal Pelves.

On the accurate determination, as far as possible, of the degree of pelvic abnormality in relation to the estimated size of the foetus depends the scientific selection of the operative procedure which offers the fairest chance both to the woman and to the foetus. Only through the deliberate election, in a given case, of a determinate operative procedure can the physician plead that he has done his whole duty by the two beings whose welfare depends on his skill. The midwifery of the present differs in many respects from that of the past. In no respect is the difference more striking than in the growing tendency to elect the proper operation before, in the face of maternal and of foetal exhaustion, it is forced upon us.

Careful inquiry into the antecedents of the patient; inspection, where need be, of the general configuration of the body,— data of this kind are essential aids in the determination of the nature of pelvic abnormality. Diseases of early life, such as rachitis and marasmus, almost inevitably leave their impress on the pelvis,—an impress which superficial pelvic examination may not reveal,—but the knowledge of which will urge the physician to bring all his skill to bear on a more careful and thorough examination of the pelvis.

The abnormalities of the female pelvis may be conveniently divided into minor and major, common and uncommon. In the United States the major deformities are rarely met with, but their determination is a far simpler matter than that of the minor deviations from the normal. It is in the latter class of cases that extreme accuracy is requisite, since at times shades of diference may turn the scale in favor of one or another operative procedure. In instances of major deformity the choice of operation will ordinarily be limited, in the presence of a foetus of average size, within a very narrow range.

The varieties of pelvic deformity and the salient characteristics of each are as follow:— *I. Justo-Major Pelvis.* The equally enlarged pelvis is of obstetric significance only in so far as it may lead to precipitate labor or to prolapse of the funis. It is not a variety of pelvic abnormality which is at all likely to call for operative interference. External pelvimetry will readily diagnosticate the condition, seeing that the diameters obtained exceed the measurements which have been stated as normal. The diagnosis, therefore, is chiefly of value as warning the attendant of the possible complications just mentioned, in order that he may be prepared to meet them. Precipitate labor may mean, for the woman, post-partum haemorrhage, inversion of the uterus, laceration of the genital tract, and prolapse of the cord may entail foetal death.

II. The Jwto-Minor Pelvis.—This form of pelvic deformity is of infrequent occurrence. The external configuration of the patient and her antecedent history may give us no clue to its presence. It is only through careful pelvimetry, external and

Fig. 7.—Generally Equally Contracted Pelvis (Justo-Minor).

internal, that the diagnosis, ordinarily, may be reached. All the diameters of the pelvis are diminished to a greater or less degree, and it is apparent how essential it is to determine the amount of diminution in order to elect the proper operative procedure in any instance where the estimated size of the foetus suggests that assistance will be needed. In general, it may be stated, that in the presence of this variety of pelvic deformity, certainly in all but the lesser grades, it is advisable to explore the pelvis manually (under anaesthesia), in order to determine, as approximately as possible, the length of the transverse and oblique diameters from the brim to the outlet. In reported instances the diminution in the diameters has amounted to an inch and over. Early recognition of this type of pelvis, therefore, might suggest the induction of premature labor: if the time for this operation had elapsed the question of choice between forceps and version might arise; in the extreme degrees of contraction the deliberate election of symphysiotomy, the Cesarean section, or of embryotomy would offer as alternatives. *III. The Flattened Pelvis.*— This abnormality of the pelvis may be met with, like the preceding, in women of normal external configuration and of healthy antecedents. It is a type of pelvis very frequently found, so much so, indeed, that many authorities rank it as the most frequent variety of deformity.

The etiological cause can rarely be definitely stated. This pelvis is found amongst all classes, the wealthy as well as the poor, amongst those subjected to privations in infancy and to toil before maturity, and those who are reared with tenderest care from the start. Pelvimetry alone, in the vast proportion of cases, will reveal the abnormality, and that its recognition is important is apparent when we recall the well-known fact that this deformity is a frequent source of the most deplorable results in childbirth.

The diagnosis of this form of pelvic deformity rests on the fact that there is narrowing in the external conjugate whilst, as a rule, the other diameters are normal. The transverse diameter may be increased; there is no pelvic asymmetry. The true conjugate measures, generally, about three inches.

From a surgical stand-point, bearing these characteristics in mind, the recognition of this form of pelvic deformity tells the physician that his aim, in case of difficulty in extraction, should be to guide the largest diameter of the foetal presenting part into the largest diameter of the pelvis. In other words, labor through this type of pelvis requires constant watchfulness on the part of the accoucheur. It is only by not trusting to nature overmuch that deplorable results, chiefly from the foetal side, may be avoided. Here, again, the question of the election of version or forceps will often be forced on the physician.

IV. The Rachitic Pelvis.—In certain sections of Europe the rachitic type of pelvis is very commonly met with. In the United States, except among our foreign-born population, this pelvis is infrequent compared with the simple flat pelvis. The external configuration of the woman may or may not suggest the presence of rachitic deformity. Inquiry into the early history of the patient will, however, generally give the requisite clue. Often, in marked instances, the appearance of the patient is characteristic; the size is dwarfed; the abdomen prominent; the gait clumsy; the sacrum is flattened externally in outline; a variable amount of spinal deviation may be present. External pelvimetry will reveal, as a rule, diminution (slight in the minor degrees of deformity) in the measurements between the crests and the spines. The external conjugate is always diminished. These results call for internal pelvimetry under anaesthesia, for the hand alone, exploring the pelvis, can give us sufficiently accurate data as to the degree of deformity. The pelvic capacity will be found to be generally limited. The pelvis is often asymmetrical.

The most marked internal change is due to the downward sinking of the sacrum, the result being approximation of the promontory to the symphysis. This antero-posterior shortening may be compensated by a slight increase in the transverse diameter, but this is not the rule in the typical rachitic pelvis. The pubic arch is generally widened. The total result of these alterations is a pelvis with contraction at the brim, whilst the outlet may be normal or slightly widened.

In the extreme degree of this deformity the approximation of the sacral promontory to the symphysis may be such as to practically divide the brim of the pelvis into two portions.

The importance of the recognition of this pelvis before labor is at once obvious. The contraction at the brim necessarily interferes with the normal engagement of the foetal presenting part. The safety of the foetus, certainly, depends therefore on the diagnosis of the deformity before long-continued efforts—leading to maternal and foetal exhaustion—at engagement have been made. Here, again, it is evident how accurate pelvic exploration before labor may teach the physician that his patient has a pelvis where the judicious election of one or another obstetric operation will redound to the safety of the child if not always, in this deformity, of the mother. In minor degrees of the deformity, even, the foetal head cannot enter the pelvic brim obliquely (as is normal). The physician, for instance, if he recognize this, may conclude that the chances for the foetus are better if he perform version and guide the largest diameters of the head through the largest of the pelvis. The brim once passed, there will be rarely difficulty in the further progress of labor in the pure rachitic type (mild) of pelvis.

The pelves, the characteristics of which have been tersely passed in review, constitute the varieties with which the practitioner will ordinarily come in contact. As a rule, these pelves, except the higher grades of rachitic deformity, rarely suggest themselves from inspection of the general configuration of the patient. The varieties which are next to be considered are of rare occurrence, certainly in English-speaking countries, and, as a rule, the appearance of the woman at once suggests the existence of pelvic deformity. Accurate pelvimetry, however, is none the less requisite, seeing that due recognition of the exact deformity may, the time being opportune, point infallibly to the necessity of the induction of premature labor or even to artificial abortion, in order to avoid at term embryotomy of the living foetus in instances where the indication for the Caesarean section is not absolute, and yet, where this operation cannot, for one or another reason, be deliberately elected.

(a) *The Transversely Contracted Pelvis.*—This type is also known as Roberts's pelvis from the fact that he first described it.

Fig. 12.—Roberts's Pelvis. The Transversely Contracted Pelvis.

It is an uncommon variety of pelvic deformity, only about thirteen instances being on record. The chief internal characteristic of this pelvis is its division into two halves anteroposteriorly. This is due to progressive narrowing of the transverse diameter from the brim to the outlet. The conjugate diameter, on the other hand, differs but little, if any, from the normal. The sinking of the sacrum into the pelvis is marked, the posterior superior spines are close together, and the iliac bones project greatly posteriorly.

(*b*) *The Kyphotic Pelvis.*—Inspection

of the patient and the antecedent history will at once suggest this deformity. The etiological cause is Pott's disease, and, according as this disease has affected one or another portion of the spinal column, the anterior deviation of the column is in the dorsal, lumbar, or sacral region.

The effect of the spinal deviation on the pelvis is variable. In general, however, the pelvis offers the following characteristics: The true conjugate is increased, the transverse diameter is lessened at the brim, diminished in the cavity, and still more so at the outlet. The sacrum is carried upward and backward; the pubic arch, as a rule, is narrowed. Where Pott's disease has developed in infancy, the total result, as regards the pelvis, is

Fig. 13.—The Kyphotic Pelvis, showing Narrowing in the Transverse Diameter and Lengthening in the Conjugate.

that its growth is arrested. This pelvis, in general, will call for the induction of premature labor, for at term the choice will almost necessarily lie between the Caesarean section and embryotomy, except in an instance of very small foetus.

(c) *The Scoliotic Pelvis.*—It is essential to differentiate two types of scoliotic pelvis,—the rachitic and the non-rachitic,—for the characteristics are markedly different.

In case of the non-rachitic scoliotic pelvis the diminution in the diameters is only exceptionally great enough to prevent delivery at term. The chief characteristics of the pelvis are: The side of the pelvis toward which the spinal column deviates is flattened to a greater or less degree. As a result one of the oblique diameters is shortened, but the other may not be altered. The pelvic inlet is chiefly the seat of contraction.

The rachitic scoliotic pelvis, on the other hand, presents alterations which differ in degree according as the rachitic

Fig. 14.—Non-Uachitic Scoliotic Skeleton. Fig. 15.—Rachitic Scoliotic Skeleton.

changes have supervened in early infancy or later. Leopold states the following as the striking characteristics of this pelvis: There is considerable shortening of the true conjugate owing to the projection forward of the sacral promontory. There is greater or less asymmetry of the pelvis according to the degree of lateral curvature of the spinal column. The symphysis of the pubes is deviated toward the side opposite the scoliosis.

At the pelvic inlet there is contraction on the side of the scoliosis and widening on the other, whilst at the outlet the reverse holds true. The antero-posterior diameter is here diminished, but more to the same degree than the true conjugate.

In the usual variety of scoliosis the dorsal vertebral column is curved toward the right, and the compensatory lumbar curve is toward the left; the pelvic capacity, therefore, is ordinarily diminished on the right. If the foetus can be borne spontaneously, it must be through the wider (left) half of the pelvis, and in a given case, where the scoliosis is right-sided, the physician in his manipulations should remember that it is within the left half of the pelvis that he can alone work.

(d) *Spondylolisthetic Pelvis.*—This pelvis results from the sliding downward of one or more of the lumbar vertebrae on the first sacral vertebra, forming a false promontory anterior to and below the true. The result is marked narrowing in the conjugate,—to such a degree, in extreme cases, that the fœtus cannot enter the pelvic cavity. The deformity was first described by Kilian. Neugebauer has most elaborately studied it, and, as a result of his analysis of forty-three cases, he reaches the conclusion that the deformity is not the result of a dyscrasia, but of the physiological weight of the trunk. This explanation, however, hardly accords with the data furnished by the museum specimens, seeing that in the majority there is evidence of the destruction of one or more of the lumbar or sacral vertebrae, suggesting Pott's disease as a causative factor.

The recognition of the deformity offers no difficulty. The contour of the lumbar spine at once suggests deformity, and digital internal pelvimetry reveals the nature of the obstruction. This form of pelvis, if detected early enough, calls for the induction of premature labor. At term the indication for the Cesarean section may be absolute.

(e) *Funnel-Shaped Pelvis.*—This variety is so exceedingly rare as to call for but passing notice. The name accurately describes the appearance of the pelvis. There is slight contraction in all the diameters at the pelvic inlet, and this narrowing increases progressively to the outlet, llecognition is easy if internal pelvimetry be not neglected, and, again, we have a pelvis where wise conservatism will counsel the induction of premature labor, for at term the choice will almost inevitably lie between the Ceesarean section and embryotomy. (/) *The Osteomalacic Pelvis.*—The disease causing this deformity usually develops after puberty, appearing, as a rule, during the gravid state. The early stages of the disease are characterized by the presence of acute pain in the limbs and pelvis, and this symptom during pregnancy should suggest the development of the disease, and should call for careful pelvic mensuration by means of the entire hand. The disease is very rare in the United States. In Italy and in certain portions of lower Germany it is frequently met with. The etiological causes are the same as those of rickets; but, except in advanced cases, the external configuration of the woman will not suggest the pelvic deformity.

The characteristics of the osteomalacic pelvis are: The bones, in general, are softened; the sacrum is small, the promontory sinking into the pelvis and approximating the symphysis. The lumbar vertebrae, in consequence, approach the pelvic brim. The rami of the pubes bend inward, the pubic angle being sharply acute and shaped like a beak. The external measurement between the iliac spines is less than normal, and that between the crests exceeds that between the spines. As a rule, the outlet of the pelvis is narrower than the inlet. Whilst the conjugate diameter may be only slightly narrowed, the transverse is considerably so at the brim and more so in the cavity and at the outlet.

In the slighter degrees of deformity

due to osteomalacia, internal pelvimetry by the entire hand is absolutely essential not alone for accurate diagnosis, but also for determining the extent to which the softened pelvic bones can be made to yield to pressure. It is very essential to determine this latter point, for on this depends the determination of delivery *per viaa naturoles* with safety to the woman. In many of the reported instances of osteomalacia the indications for Caesarean section have been absolute. Of 72 cases collected by Litzmann, 38 could not be delivered naturally. It is also to be remembered that the disease is aggravated in successive pregnancies.

If recognized in time, the osteomalacic pelvis calls for the induction of premature labor; in aggravated instances, for artificial abortion. If determined only at term, whilst the pelvis may yield sufficiently to allow of the delivery of the foetus, in the vast proportion of cases the physician will be called upon to elect either embryotomy or the Cesarean section,—here, as always prior to maternal exhaustion, the result of ineffectual efforts at delivery.

(!/) *The Oblique Ovate Pelvis.*—This form of pelvic deformity was first described by Naegele. As a rule, the woman offers no external signs. The broad characteristics of the pelvis are the diminution of one oblique diameter associated with ankylosis of one of the sacro-iliac synchondroses. The pelvis is asymmetrical, one side of the sacrum is lacking in development, and the bone is pushed toward the affected side. The pubic symphysis is obliquely opposite the sacrum. The arch of the pubes is narrowed. The true conjugate is, as a rule, longer than normal; the transverse is narrowed at the brim, and this narrowing increases progressively toward the outlet. Pelvic mensuration of the lateral halves will reveal the asymmetry.

In aggravated instances the rule as regards the external configuration will not hold. The woman limps, one hip is higher than the other, and deviation of the pubes is marked. In such an instance the following measurements, which are the same in a normal pelvis and shorter on the affected side in the oblique ovate pelvis, should be taken as assisting in diagnosis: From the tuberosities of the ischium to the opposed posterior superior spines of the ilium; from the anterior superior to the opposite posterior superior spines; from the spinous process of the last lumbar vertebra to the anterior superior spines. These measurements may readily be taken with the pelvimeter. The oblique ovate pelvis is of not infrequent occurrence. The necessity of recognition is apparent from the statement that in a series of instances collected by Litzmann, 22 out of 28 women died and out of 41 children 31 were lost. Such results are explainable alone on the assumption that the variety of deformity was not recognized before term. This pelvis calls strictly for the induction of premature labor in order to avoid the choice at term between the Caesarean section and embryotomy. Only exceptionally, and then in the lesser degree of the deformity, can spontaneous labor at term occur, or will, at this time, version or the forceps be safe for the woman. Symphysiotomy is contraindicated.

(7f) *Pelves Deformed by Tumors.*—The presence of tumors within the pelvic cavity obviously interferes with the progress of labor and may even render delivery by the natural passages impossible. These tumors may be bony projections (exostoses), osteosarcomata, carcinomata, fibroids of the uterus, ovarian cysts; such, at least, are the common varieties. According to the size of these tumors will vary the obstetric operation requisite for delivery. Ordinarily their presence may be detected only by exploration of the pelvis; hence a further reason for the rule already dwelt upon,—the necessity for examining the pelvis of every gravid woman at an early date of gestation. Such a rule, if ordinarily followed, and if its necessity be recognized by every woman, will, time and again, result in the choice of a minor operative procedure,—such as artificial abortion or the induction of premature labor, in instances where, if the woman be only examined at term, the indication for the Caesarean section may be absolute. Further, in case of pediculated fibroids, for instance, the risk resulting from impaction within the brim may be avoided where the woman is seen in the early stage of gestation, seeing that, at times, manipulation in the proper position—the knee-chest—may enable the physician to push the growth above the brim; and in case of an ovarian cyst, for instance, the advisability of abdominal section for its removal might well be forced on the physician.

The osseous, cancerous, sarcomatous tumors which spring from the walls of the pelvic cavity will, as a rule, if not detected till term, call for embryotomy or for the Cesarean section, possibly for the Porro operation. It must be recognized as unscientific, to say the least, to attempt delivery by either forceps or version where the foetus is estimated at average size and the tumor narrows the pelvis sufficiently to warrant the assumption that delivery without mutilation is problematical.

Aside from the death of or injuries inflicted upon the child by attempts at forceps extraction, the trauma the woman would necessarily be subjected to is a distinct contra-indication.

From this analysis of the salient characteristics of deformed pelves it is apparent how helpless the practitioner may be, at the term of gestation or when labor is advanced, if, for one or another reason, he has neglected or it has been impracticable to estimate the capacity of the pelvis either at an early stage of gestation or before the onset of labor.

Without the data obtainable. through pelvimetry and exploration of the pelvis, it is impossible to elect the obstetric operation, where one is demanded, which best subserves in a given case the interest of the two beings whose safety depends on the acquired knowledge and expertness of the accoucheur. In practical obstetrics, the forceps, for example, is too often used in instances where accurate pelvimetry will teach that it is contra-indicated. The major obstetric procedures are too frequently delayed until maternal and foetal exhaustion is imminent or present. The facts on which stress has been laid teach the necessity of deliberate election of every obstetric operation, and it is from this stand-point that these operations will be considered.

3 CHAPTER II. ARTIFICIAL ABORTION AND THE INDUCTION OF PREMATURE LABOR.

The term "abortion" is applied to instances where the uterus is emptied of the product of conception either spontaneously or artificially before this product has reached that stage of development when it is fitted for extra-uterine life. Artificial abortion, therefore, is performed purely in the interests of the woman. Premature labor, on the other hand, when induced, carries witli it the assumption that the foetus is capable of surviving apart from the mother,—that is to say, that this foetus has reached what is termed the viable age. This operation, then, is resorted to both in the interests of mother and child, although ordinarily those of the former chiefly urge the physician to resort to it. The induction of premature labor is, in general, an elective operation; artificial abortion is usually forced on the physician. The factors calling for the one operation are usually different from those calling for the other, and the method of procedure also differs. It is useful, therefore, to consider the subjects apart.

(«) Artificial Abortion.

The diseases and anomalies which justify artificial abortion are: 1. Advanced pulmonary and cardiac disease. 2. The pernicious vomiting of pregnancy. 3. Renal disease. 4. Pernicious anaemia. 5. Chorea. 6. Absolute pelvic contraction or occlusion of the genital tract by tumors, etc. 7. Irreducible displacements of the uterus. 8. Haemorrhage from placenta praevia, hydatid mole, etc.

Bearing in mind strictly the fact that artificial abortion is performed purely in the interests of the woman, we will consider these indications *seriatim*. 1. *Advanced Pulmonary and Cardiac Disease.*—At a glance it is apparent what an untoward effect gestation, if allowed to advance, must have on the life-limit of a woman in an advanced stage of phthisis or with serious cardiac lesion.

The vital force of the woman is being actively expended in fighting the disease which shortly will kill her when, in addition, the extra burden of supporting foetal growth for nine months is thrown upon her. If such a woman be allowed to go to term, even if she can withstand the strain of pregnancy and of labor, the duration of her remnant of life has unquestionably been shortened, and she will rarely have the satisfaction of leaving behind her a healthy babe. Wise and justifiable conservatism, therefore, counsels the artificial arrest of pregnancy as soon as detected, in case of advanced phthisis and of a cardiac lesion which has progressed to the stage of dilatation.

The indication may be said to be absolute in the former instance; in the latter only when the heart has begun to dilate, since otherwise the physiological cardiac hypertrophy of pregnancy will enter as a compensatory factor, and enable the woman to reach term with safety, and, likely enough, not deteriorated in general health.

2. *The Pernicious Vomiting of Pregnane)/.*—This indication may be called absolute only after the recognized general and local remedies have been tried. Rectification of a uterine displacement, applications of solutions of nitrate of silver to the cervix, digital or instrumental dilatation of the cervix, regulation of the diet and of the function of the intestinal canal, the internal administration of drugs (oxalate of cerium in large doses, ingluvin, minim doses of ipecac or of phenic acid),— such, briefly stated, are the chief measures on which dependence may be placed for the relief of pernicious vomiting. Only after such means have been tested does artificial abortion suggest itself as justifiable. It should then be deliberately elected. The physician should not wait until the emaciation is extreme, the pulse is rapid, and the fever of exhaustion sets in. On the occurrence of phenomena of exhaustion, the operation may fail in its object,—the saving of maternal life,—and generally emptying of the uterus is postponed too late. The fact that the vomiting, even when of the so-called pernicious type, in many instances ceases spontaneously at the third month, whilst a cause for hope, should never blind the physician to such a degree as to lead him to expectancy overlong. Whilst, as a rule, artificial abortion, under this indication, is rarely called for, it is safer not to wait until the vital forces of the woman are at too low an ebb.

3. *Renal Disease.*—The co-existence of renal disease and of pregnancy is most unfortunate. Aside from the strong probability of the development of eclampsia, if the pregnancy be allowed to continue, the extra wear on the kidneys associated with gestation inevitably tends to shorten the woman's life if she be allowed to go to term. This in particular holds true of the parenchymatous form of nephritis. In a given case, if under absolute milk diet and the administration of iron and diuretics the amount of albumin in the urine do not decrease, artificial abortion should be resorted to. In the event of betterment from the side of the kidneys, then, under constant watchfulness, the woman might be tided over until the child is viable, and often to term. 4. *Pernicious Anaemia.*—This indication will rarely offer for the reason that the affection is only exceptionally met with, and then conception is a rarity owing to the lack of function of the ovaries. In the event, however, of pregnancy supervening on this depraved condition of the blood, artificial abortion is justifiable as soon as it becomes apparent that the anaemia, notwithstanding the recognized remedies, is becoming deeper. To wait longer is to aggravate the disease, only to obtain a foetus incapable of extra-uterine life. 5. *Chorea.*—Pregnancy has a deleterious influence on chorea. In all the reported instances the choreic movements have become aggravated often to an extreme degree. Nature sometimes asserts herself and abortion is spontaneous. On the other hand, it cannot be positively predicated that emptying the uterus will modify the chorea favorably. The indication, therelore, for artificial abortion is not an absolute one. The operation should be

resorted to only in extreme instances, and then only in the hope that it may prove a remedial measure. Barnes's statistics prove that gravid choi-eic women often die of the disease, and that the foetus rarely survives. It should further be remembered that in a lew recorded instances chorea associated with pregnancy has merged into one or another variety of insanity. 6. *Absolute Pelvic Contraction or Occlusion of the Genital Tract by Tumors, etc.*—By absolute pelvic contraction is understood that degree of pelvic deformity which will not even permit of the induction of premature labor with viable child. This will be amply considered when the subject of premature labor is discussed. As soon as determined, artificial abortion is indicated in order to save the woman the risks of the alternative operations at term,—the CEesarean section or the Porro.

Until the results from these operations are of such a nature as to prove no greater mortality rates than that after abortion, the duty of the physician, unless the woman deliberately elects the major operations, is to empty the uterus. The same view may be taken of instances of cicatricial contraction of the vagina of such high degree as to preclude the successful induction of premature labor. The tumors which come under consideration, aside from exostoses, are fibroids in the lower uterine segment, epithelioma of the cervix, impacted ovarian cysts. Exostoses, if sufficiently prominent to occlude the pelvis to a degree inconsistent with the successful induction of premature labor, will always call for artificial abortion unless, again, the woman elects the Cesarean section at term; fibroids in the lower segment of the uterus do not, as a rule, interfere with the development of the uterus to the term of foetal viability, at any rate; but at this date, and later, the choice will necessarily lie between enucleation of the fibroid *per vaginam* before delivery can be effected or else the Cesarean section or the Porro. Enucleation of a fibroid by the vagina is at best a formidable operation, and becomes all the more so in the presence of the vascularity associated with pregnancy. To say nothing of the risk of septicaemia during the puerperium, the safety of the woman is best subserved by emptying the uterus at an early stage, unless, again, in full view of its risks, she elects the alternative operations at term. It is understood, of course, that an ovarian cyst impacted in the pelvis cannot be removed through abdominal section without first emptying the uterus; therefore, the proper course to pursue is to induce abortion, and at one and the same time to remove the cyst by one or another of the recognized methods. Epithelioma of the uterus, whenever discovered, should be removed either by high amputation or by vaginal hysterectomy. In either event the gestation will be interrupted; so that artificial abortion is forced on the physician, and not elected. Advanced carcinoma of the lower uterine segment, when complicated by pregnancy, becomes all the more serious the longer the gestation is allowed to continue. The chief risk the woman runs is that from sudden profuse haemorrhage; but, seeing that the woman may be made more comfortable by a partial operation, this should be resorted to even though it interrupt gestation. At term delivery *per vias naturales* might be possible without fatal result to the woman; but this being problematical, active interference is justifiable before the child is viable. Fortunately women with advanced carcinoma rarely conceive.

It is a recognized surgical rule, today, to remove an ovarian cyst as soon as it is discovered. If pregnancy co-exist, ovariotomy may be performed and the gestation not interrupted. This is exceptional in the favorable case, when the tumor is not impacted in the pelvis. In the latter instance the maternal chances are better if the uterus be first emptied *lege arils,* and the ovariotomy be performed afterward. Obviously the physician should be on his guard lest, during the process of abortion, the cyst rupture. Puncture of the cyst by the vagina as an elective measure cannot too strongly be condemned. Whilst such a measure will diminish the size of the tumor, and thus, perhaps, enable the gestation to advance nearly or to term, with resulting viable foetus, puncture, however aseptically performed, carries with it the risk of suppuration of the cyst, in which event neither abortion nor ovariotomy might avail to save the woman. Obviously, where the obstructing tumors are so large as to interfere with access to the uterine cavity, it ceases to be a question of even artificial abortion, and the physician is called upon to decide upon the relative risks of interference surgically with the tumor before or at term. Where the risk is equal the latter period should, of course, be selected, since the child is then given a chance.

7. *Irreducible Displacements of the Uterus.*—No displacement of the uterus uncomplicated by adhesions must be considered irreducible so as to require artificial abortion until replacement under anaesthesia, with the woman in the kneechest position, has failed. Simpler methods are, of course, first to be tested. Impaction of the gravid uterus below the promontory of the sacrum may simulate an adherent uterus; but if the woman assume the knee-chest position and the cervix be drawn downward by means of a tenaculum inserted into the anterior lip, reposition may, as a rule, be effected if the displacement be uncomplicated. In an instance of this nature, if seen before the third month, emptying of the uterus will rarely be called for. It is the adherent fundus which generally will give rise to trouble. Unquestionably, in many of these instances, the adhesions stretch and enable the uterus to rise above the brim; but where this does not occur, gentle attempts at manual stretching of the adhesions having failed, artificial abortion should be resorted to before the uterus, developing asymmetrically,—in case spontaneous abortion do not occur,—causes grave symptoms from the side of the bladder, possibly leading to rupture of the organ.

8. *Haemorrhage.*—The slight discharge of blood which not uncommonly complicates the early months of pregnancy will never call for artificial abortion. Rest in bed with appropriate reme-

dies—such as the viburnum prunifolinm and, perhaps, an opiate; removal of the cause, such as a small submucous polyp—will, as a rule, suffice to check what at times is simply an attempt at periodical menstruation. It is the haemorrhage met with between the third and sixth months of gestation which may warrant abortion. Haemorrhage at this period should always suggest a low attachment of the placenta, and, when profuse enough to threaten maternal exhaustion, it is conservative to empty the uterus rather than to endeavor to tide over the patient until the fœtus has attained viability.

Such, briefly outlined, are the complications of early pregnancy which chiefly will call for artificial abortion. This operation should never be determined upon without the advice of a consultant. The risk to the woman where the operation is carefully performed is slight, presumably always slighter than that she is subject to if the gestation be not interrupted; but no physician, except in strict emergency, should induce an abortion without the support of one or more consultants. He will thus be amply protected against scandal and legal process, should either arise.

In view of the fact that artificial abortion is an operation which is forced upon the physician, when the indication presents, the object is to empty the uterus as rapidly as is consistent with the welfare of the woman. The method of procedure about to be described is peculiarly applicable to gestation which has not advanced beyond the third month. After this period, the fœtus and its adnexa being larger, and fuller dilatation of the cervical canal being therefore requisite, the method to be described under the subject of the induction of premature labor is to be selected.

The administration of so-called abortifacients and resort to electricity are proposed methods for the induction of abortion which are so problematical in their results as not to be worthy of trial. Tamponing the vagina, associated with the administration of ergot, was a method formerly greatly in vogue. It should be rejected, however, because it is slow in action, uncertain in its results, and difficult to maintain aseptically. The sponge tent for dilating the cervix cannot be too strongly condemned, on the ground that the chances of sepsis following its use are very great. It should ever be borne in mind that the operation is performed in the interest of the woman, and that the one risk the physician subjects her to is sepsis.

OPERATION FOR THE INDUCTION OF ABORTION.

The instruments strictly requisite are: A steel-branched uterine dilator, a uterine dull curette, an ovum forceps, an intrauterine irrigating tube, the finger. These instruments should be carefully sterilized.

The intestinal canal should be thoroughly emptied by enema, and the bladder by catheter. The external genitals and the vagina must be thoroughly asepticized. Douching will not accomplish this. Both the genitals and the vagina should be scrubbed with soap and water, and then washed with a 2-per-cent. solution of creolin or a 1 to 5000 solution of bichloride of mercury. Thus alone may the rugosities of the vagina be rendered aseptic. If the operator prefer continuous irrigation during his manipulations the creolin solution answers admirably, since it will not injure the instruments and will not poison the patient. The hands of the operator and of his assistant should be scrupulously scrubbed with soap and water, and then carefully washed in a solution of bichloride of mercury. These details are called for in order to avoid septic infection of the patient,—the risk, we would repeat, which the woman is subjected to. As a rule, it is desirable to anaesthetize the patient. The operation, when resorted to at all, must be thorough, and it is difficult to secure this if the patient be struggling and complaining. The patient is placed upon the table in the left lateral or dorsal position, according to the preference of the operator. We prefer the dorsal position because all the necessary steps are best followed in this position, and because, furthermore, the uterus is under better control.

A speculum is inserted into the vagina, and, the cervix having been exposed, a tenaculum is inserted into the anterior cervical lip to steady the uterus.

The steel dilator is passed into the cervix beyond the internal os, and the canal is slowly stretched to the extent of an inch and a half to two inches. The cervical muscle is made to yield to the applied pressure; the aim is not to rapture the cervix. Owing to the hyperemia and softening of the cervix, which, as a rule, is present even in the early months of pregnancy, dilatation to this extent will ordinarily be possible. The instruments are then to be removed, and the next step is the extraction of the ovum.

The best of all instruments for the loosening of the ovum, the breaking up of the foetus, and for the removal of the *debris* is the aseptic finger. It is sentient, and therefore it is less likely to do harm than any instrument. We are operating to protect the interests of the woman, and, therefore, must take every precaution to see that these interests are not endangered. In the average case of abortion under the third month it is possible to empty the uterus by the finger alone, provided the physician proceeds as follows: The woman should be anaesthetized. The fundus of the uterus is grasped through the abdominal wall, and the organ is depressed deeply into the pelvic cavity in the axis of the inferior strait. The other hand is introduced into the vagina, and the index finger is inserted to the fundus of the uterus, slowly, in order to obtain greater dilatation than has followed the use of the dilator. The ovum is then carefully peeled from its connection with the uterus. Up to the second month of gestation it may ordinarily be removed in its entirety. Beyond this period it is usually necessary to break up the ovum by the intra-uterine finger, and this may be accomplished without great difficulty, provided the external hand firmly controls and steadies the uterus.

In instances where it is not possible to depress the uterus sufficiently to enable the finger (the hand being in the vagina) to reach the site of the ovum, the long uterine curette takes the place of the finger. The instrument, however, should be used simply to loosen the connection of the ovum with the uterus, the after-extraction being accomplished either by means of the ovum-forceps or by the finger. The manipulation is as follows: The curette seeks to penetrate between the ovum and the uterine wall, the external hand being conscious of and thus indirectly controlling the action of the instrument. When dislodged in this manner, if the finger cannot complete removal, the ovum-forceps should be used to grasp and to extract it.

The haemorrhage from these manipulations is, as a rule, considerable, but the external hand grasping the uterus may soon cause efficient contraction. When satisfied that the uterus has been thoroughly emptied, a J-drachm of ergot or 10 minims of ergotole should be injected into the nates, the intra-uterine tube should be inserted into the cavity of the uterus and the organ washed out either with a 1 to 5000 solution of bichloride of mercury or with a 3-per-cent. solution of creolin. The last step, and we believe a most important step, is the insertion to the fundus of a sterilized-gauze drain.

The object of this drain is twofold: At times, owing to

Fljf. 27.—Intra-uterine Dressing Forceps.

flexion at the level of the internal os, drainage from the uterine cavity is imperfect and the retained secretions might give rise to septic symptoms; furthermore, no matter how exact our asepsis, an error in technique may creep in, and, if local sepsis should develop, we want above all tilings free external drainage, in order to avoid, as far as is possible, extension to the Fallopian tubes. This drain, therefore, is prophylactic in its aim. It can do no harm, and it may be the means of preventing serious damage.

The steps detailed will answer for the induction of abortion and for its completion in the average case under the fourth month. Occasionally, however, the cervix is rigid, and then the steel-branched dilator and the finger cannot secure ampleenough dilatation. In such an event-many practitioners resort to tents; but for the reason already stated and again emphasized, that the sponge tent cannot be rendered aseptic, we emphatically condemn this agent (including as well all other forms of tent), and we commend the following procedure: The external genitals and the vagina having been rendered aseptic in the manner we have dwelt upon, the cervix is exposed through a speculum and steadied by a tenaculum. As much dilatation as possible is secured by the steel-branched dilator, and then the cervical canal and the lower uterine segment is packed by means of the intra-uterine dressing forceps with sterilized gauze. At the end of from six to eight hours the gauze may be removed, when, as a rule, the cervical canal will be found sufficiently patulous for the finger or else the cervical tissues have been sufficiently softened by the gauze to enable the steel-branched dilator to act efficiently. The further steps are similar to those already detailed.

There remain for consideration those instances where the cervical canal is not accessible to the dilator, owing, as a rule, to the marked retroversion of the uterus with or without adhesions. It has been recommended, in such instances, to puncture the uterus through the rectum, the object being to tap the amniotic sac, which procedure will result in spontaneous abortion. This method should never be resorted to, owing to the absolute certainty of carrying products of infection into the uterus. The rectum cannot be asepticized as may the vagina. The aim of the method will be as well subserved by tapping through the vagina, care being taken to avoid any large vessels and also the ureteral triangle. Very rarely will such a step be necessary, however, and if resorted to the method must be called an uncertain one. In the nice of an emergency suggesting it, it is wise to weigh the alternative step,—abdominal section, the breaking up of the adhesions, and reposition, *per abdominem,* of the uterus.

Artificial abortion, if performed aseptically, and if elected before the woman is at too low an ebb from the affection indieating the operation, ought not to have a mortality rate. Haemorrhage we may control; sepsis is avoidable by the steps of the operation we have advocated; shock need be feared only when the physician sees the patient too late or trusts to expectancy overlong. The after-treatment of cases where the physician has been called upon to induce abortion is similar to that which is applicable to the puerperium after delivery at term. The woman should remain in bed for about a week, not necessarily in the recumbent position, however. If there be no contra-indication from the side of the heart, and if the disease which called for the induction of abortion will permit, it is decidedly advantageous for the patient to sit up in bed according to her fancy, for thus the vagina drains to better advantage.

If the operation has been performed aseptically, there will be no call for either vaginal or intra-uterine douching. Where a gauze drain has been inserted into the uterine cavity, it may be removed at.the end of sixty hours; and if there be no evidence of local sepsis, it need not be re-inserted. If, notwithstanding all our aseptic precautions, sepsis develop, its surgical treatment will be in accordance with the rules to be emphasized in the chapter dealing with the surgery of the pathological puerperium.

(b) The Induction Of Premature Labor. Obviously, the indications for the induction of abortion hold with equal, if not greater, stringency in case of the induction of premature labor. The object to be attained, however, is twofold. Both the interests of the fcetus and of the woman are to be considered. Exceptionally, as will be noted, those of the former alone call for the operation. From the side of both the woman and of the child, the chief indications for the induction of premature labor are: 1. Contracted pelves. 2. Haemorrhage. 3. Eclampsia.

From the stand-point of the child alone the indication offers where, in a previous labor, the foetus has died a short time before term as a result, frequently, of disease of the placenta, such as fatty degeneration. Here, by electing premature labor in a succeeding pregnancy a few weeks before term, at a period when, from the decrease in foetal movements, it may be inferred that death is imminent, the physician may succeed in obtaining a living child.

1. *Induction of Premature Labor in Case of Deformity of the Pelvis.*—Deformity of the pelvis of varying grade is by far the most frequent indication for the induction of premature labor. The aim is a most beneficent one, seeing that the major obstetrical operations—the Caesarean section, symphysiotomy, and embryotomy—are thus often avoided. As Robert Barnes, with a certain amount of truth, puts it, spontaneous labor may supersede the forceps, the forceps may supersede version, version craniotomy, and the Caesarean section may be eliminated. Whether it is desirable or not that craniotomy should supersede the Cesarean section will be considered later, as also the effect of the resuscitation of symphysiotomy.

In the instances under consideration, the problem for the physician to solve is most complex. He must determine as accurately as possible the term of gestation, in order to speak with any degree of authority in regard to the chances of viability of the child. He must estimate the probable size of the foetus in relation to the degree of pelvic contraction in a given case. He must bear in mind the degree of molding to which the diameters of the foetal head are susceptible within safe limits. He must, lastly, ever be conscious of the fact that in deferring the operation overlong in the interest of the child he may be increasing the risks which the woman runs. It is thus apparent how difficult it is to select just the right time for the induction of premature labor from an elective standpoint.

The determination of the stage of gestation so as to insure foetal viability is not a simple matter. In almost every instance there is likely to be a margin in error of at least a fortnight. Where the exact date of the cessation of menstruation can be ascertained, the rule of adding seven days and counting back three months, in order to approximate the term of gestation, is exact enough only in the lesser grades of pelvic deformity; for here, if the error of a fortnight creep in, at best the child has not passed the seven and a half months of gestation. Where the interests of the child, on the other hand, demand the induction of premature labor at the seventh month, at least, the difficulty in determining this date might lead us to resort to the operation before the term of viability or else beyond it, when, in either event, the operation, so far as the child were concerned, would be a failure. The two hundred and twentieth day of gestation may be taken as the lowest limit when, with the improved means at our disposal (the *couveuse,* or incubator), a chance of the child being reared exists. Error in our data below this period may be taken as being fatal to the child. Not only, therefore, is it essential to obtain as accurately as possible the date of the cessation of the last menstruation, but also that of quickening. The first sensation of foetal motion occurs from three to three and a half months after conception, in some cases not till the fourth month. Here, again, is a chance of error of a fortnight. But, by weighing the probable date of conception against the date of perception of foetal motion and comparing this with the height of the uterus above the pelvic brim, the physician is, at any rate, unlikely to err against the term of viability. It will be remembered, of course, that the general statement of the height of the uterus at various stages of gestation is subject to modification in the presence of a contracted pelvis. Whilst, normally, the fundus of the uterus is on a level with the umbilicus at the sixth month of gestation, and about two fingers' breadth above this at the seventh month, in case of contraction chiefly at the pelvic brim these relative situations will be a trifle higher. Thus, at the sixth month the fundus may occupy the position which normally it would at the seventh.

Having determined as accurately as possible the date of conception, the next factor is the estimation of the size of the foetus which must pass through the given contracted pelvis. The size of the foetus can, of course, only be relatively estimated. The best guide at our disposal is that furnished by Ahlfeld, and the value of this guide at best is very limited. From extended study, Ahlfeld concluded that the long axis of the foetus lying flexed in the uterus is nearly half the entire length of the foetus when extended. To determine the axis *in utero* of the foetus, one arm of a pelvimeter is placed in the vagina in contact with the foetal presenting part, and the other arm is placed on the abdomen at the site of the fundus over the other end of the fœtus. Multiplying the obtained measurement by two, the total length of the foetus is obtained. According to Ahlfeld, the length of the extended foetus bears a certain definite relation to the period of gestation. Thus: From the 38th to the 40th week of gestation the length of the intra-uterine foetal axis varies from 9J inches to 10. The total length of the foetus, therefore, is about 20 inches. From the 35th to the 38th week the intra-uterine axis varies between 8f and 9J inches. The length of the foetus is 181 to 191 inches. From the 30th to the 35th week the intra-uterine length varies from 8j to 8? inches, and the total length of the fetus is 16 to 18 inches. From the 25th to the 30th week the intra-uterine length varies from 7 to 8 inches, and the mean total length of the fetus is about 15 inches.

Ahlfeld further determined that this length of the fetus stood in the following relation to the weight:—

The data furnished by these researches of Ahlfeld, whilst only of approximate value in estimating the size of the foetus, are still of great assistance in determining the period at which labor should be induced. An important factor lacking, however, is the average size of the fetal head at various stages of gestation. The diameter of the foetal head of the greatest importance is the biparietal. As the result of many measurements made by Budin, Tarnier, Stolz, and others, the average length of this diameter at various stages of gestation is: at term, about 3f inches; at 8 months, about 3.4 inches; at 8 months, about 3.2 inches; at 7 J months, about 2.96 inches; at 7 months, about 2.75 inches.

The foetal head, further, may be safely compressed to the extent of about 0.4 inch. Remembering this degree of safe compressibility, having estimated the size of the foetus and the stage of gestation, the next important element in the problem is the determination of the degree of pelvic deformity present. Before passing, however, to renewed reference to this, we will state the method of estimating the adaptability of the foetal presenting part to the pelvic canal which answers every purpose for private practice, and which commends itself, also, on account of its simplicity.

As long as the foetal presenting part can enter the pelvic brim, obviously the time for the induction of premature labor may be deferred; but just as soon as the presenting part engages with difficulty, the time is ripe for interference.

Every week, therefore, the physician should examine his patient for the purpose of determining the above fact. Introducing one or more fingers into the vagina, he presses the fundus of the uterus downward in the axis of the pelvic inlet and the fingers in the vagina are able to appreciate the ease with which the presenting part adapts itself to the pelvic brim. If need be, the patient should be examined under anaesthesia. (See Fig. 2, Plate III.)

By reference to Chapter I the method of determining the pelvic diameters and the characteristics of the chief varieties of pelvic contraction will be recalled. Taking the length of the conjugate of the brim as our guide, seeing that it is the internal diameter of the pelvis which alone can be determined with any degree of accuracy, and remembering that in a given case the capacity of the pelvis may be approximately estimated best by examination by the entire hand under anaesthesia, we may, with Charpentier, formulate the following general rules, which are the result of an extended study of the reports of numerous maternities and clinics:—

Tf the conjugate is at least 3i inches, the biparietal diameter of the foetal head at term being 3f inches (compressible to the extent of about 0.4 inch), then, in multiparas, labor should be induced between 8i to *8* months, according to the estimated size of the foetus and the difficulty in delivery offered by former labors. In primiparae, since, in general, the child is smaller, it is safe to wait till a week before term. Where the conjugate is 3.35 inches premature labor, both in the multipara and in the primipara, should be induced at 8 to *8h* months. Where the conjugate is 3.12 inches, labor is to be induced between 8 and *8h* months at least. Where the conjugate is 2.95 inches, labor is to be induced between 7 and 8 months. Where the conjugate is 2.75 inches, labor is to be induced between 7 months and 7 months and 3 weeks. Where the conjugate is *21* to 2.36 inches, labor must be induced as near the seventh month as practicable, and certainly no later than 7£ months. Below 2.36 inches the indication for the induction of premature labor does not exist. To resort to it would necessarily entail an embryotomy, and this carries risk to the mother and subserves not the child. At this point, then, the indication for artificial abortion in contracted pelves begins.

It is to be remembered that the figures just given hold good only for the foetus estimated to be of the average size, and for a pelvis which ranks under the flat type or, possibly, the generally contracted type. The prognosis for the child is better, under the measurements given, if the pelvis be of the former variety than if it be of the latter. In general, of course, the special type of pelvis will alter the indication. All that we aim to do here is to state the general indications which serve as guides in the election of the period at which premature labor should be induced in the face of pelvic deformity. It is impossible to lay down special rules, since each case must be studied from its special stand-point.

2. *Haemorrhage as an Indication for the Induction of Premature Labor.*—Haemorrhage occurring after the fourth month of gestation should always awaken the suspicion of placenta praevia. There is little agreement amongst obstetrical writers as to the advisability of inducing premature labor on the appearance of the first haemorrhage due to faulty implantation of the placenta. A careful study of this question, in the light chiefly of the mo e modern statistical data, warrants the following statements, which assist in reaching a conclusion sound in practice, seeing that it takes account of the interests both of the woman and the child. As has been noted under the subject of artificial abortion, in rare instances the haemorrhage due to faulty insertion of the placenta occurs as early as the fifth month of gestation. As a rule, however, it is within the six weeks preceding term that haemorrhage appears. Usually the first haemorrhage is not profuse enough to endanger either the woman or the child. It may be taken, however, as nature's danger signal, warning the alert physician that a second haemorrhage may at any time occur, and in such amount that not alone will the child probably die before delivery, but that the woman as well will be seriously endangered. Instances of this nature are extreme ones, but in no given case can it be predicted that such will not be the issue of the second haemorrhage. Unquestionably, through enforced rest in bed, the woman may often be tided to term and delivery be safely accomplished for the child as well as for the woman; but even during rest in bed profuse haemorrhage may occur, and this too at a time when the physician may not be in ready reach of the woman. All authorities are agreed that the excessive maternal mortality of the past was due, in part, to faulty methods of treatment, in part to delay in resort to active measures. The maternal mortality has varied from 32 to 9 per cent, and the infantile from 50 to 85 per cent. The modern method of treatment has given a maternal mortality, in the hands of various observers, of from 1 to 4 per cent., whilst even the infantile mortality has been lowered. The facts, then, at our disposal prove clearly that by any and all methods the child surfers excessively, whilst for the woman there is a choice in method.

The question may he summed up as follows: The risk to the woman increases progressively to term after the first lnemorrhage. On the occurrence of this hemorrhage the child is viable. Renewed haemorrhage simply risks viability. The interests of the child, therefore, are not subserved by expectancy. Those of the woman are actually imperiled. The teaching is sound, therefore, which says: On the occurrence of the first haemorrhage, whether profuse or not, elect the induction of premature labor. The earlier the haemorrhage, the greater the chance of the placenta being implanted centrally. It is central implantation which at term subjects the woman to the greatest risks and holds out but very slim chance for the child.

3. *Eclampsia as an Indication for the Induction of Premature Labor.*—Absolute statement in regard to this indication is not wise owing to the very just diversity of opinion amongst experienced obstetricians. To reach an approximately accurate conclusion it will be necessary to sharply differentiate the instances where eclampsia seems imminent and those where convulsions have developed.

Albuminuria is an almost constant forerunner and accompaniment of eclampsia. Such, at least, is the rule with but rare exceptions. The albuminuria may or may not be dependent on organic renal disease, and in the latter instance it may or may not lead to organic disease. The question, therefore, which the physician has chiefly to face is the immediate risk to mother and child if pregnancy be allowed to progress to term, remembering that in no given case can it be predicated that the emptying of the uterus will ward off the convulsions, and also that the interference with gestation may excite convulsions. The problem, it is evident, is most complex. Still, the following considerations help toward its solution.

In the vast majority of instances, the development of eclampsia leads to premature labor. If we do not shut our eyes, then, to nature's teachings, it seems wise, in the presence of eclampsia, to resort to such measures as will hasten the emptying of the uterus instead of to such as will tend to protract the gestation. The latter course, certainly, will avail naught to the child, for its life is directly imperiled by the first eclampsic attack, and, should it survive this and labor not occur spontaneously, its chances of living through further attacks are all the less. As regards the woman, if spontaneous premature labor do not occur during the first attack, experience teaches that the liability to further attacks is greater if the uterus has not been emptied than where it has. The first attack exhausts the woman, if it do no more. The second attack adds to her exhaustion and may kill. Therefore, in the presence of eclampsia it may be stated that, in general, nothing is gained by endeavoring to protract gestation and everything may be lost. One of the recognized methods of treatment of eclampsia is deep anaesthesia protracted, if need be, for hours. During this anaesthesia resort to the measures we shall shortly consider will empty the uterus possibly of a live child, for at the period of gestation under consideration the child is viable; otherwise it becomes a question of artificial abortion,—a subject already considered.

AVhere convulsions are imminent, there is even greater diversity of opinion as to the advisability of inducing labor. Whilst apparently imminent, they may never occur; the induction of premature labor may not ward them off; indeed, the measures necessary for induction may provoke convulsions. In the face of this fair statement of fact, what ground is there for advocating the operation *l* Supposing that, in spite of resort to the recognized methods of treatment of albuminuria, in particular absolute milk diet combined with iron, the albumin increases in amount, headache and visual disturbances appear, dropsy to a greater or less degree sets in. The woman has readied the seventh month; the child is viable, and the foetal heart certifies that it is alive. It may be safely predicated that the chances are that this woman will have eclampsia before or at term, daring labor or afterward. If she do before the onset or the completion of labor, the child's chances of survival are very slight. Meantime the woman risks aggravation in the renal symptoms and condition, disturbances of vision more or less permanent, puerperal mania, and puerperal paralysis. Now, if the operation of inducing premature labor be elected at the period under consideration, the child's chances arc better even if, as the result of the manipulations, eclampsia is induced; for, as already stilted, in the presence of eclampsia rapid emptying of the uterus is advisable. As for the woman, medical and dietetic treatment having failed to arrest the progress of albuminuria (the usual forerunner of eclampsia), the induction of premature labor may save her the complications just enumerated, to any and all of which she is liable if the pregnancy is allowed to go to term. Should eclampsia develop as the result of the necessary manipulations, labor having been started it may be more quickly ended than if emptying of the uterus is forced upon the physician by the spontaneous occurrence of convulsions.

As the case has been stated, therefore, the immediate and the remote welfare of the woman calls for the induction of premature labor in instances where the development of eclampsia is feared; and this fact should outweigh the argument, from the side of the child, that its chances of survival are less the earlier before term it is born, whether spontaneously or artificially. To be born in the midst or at the expiration of an eclampsic seizure at the eighth month or at term imperils its existence fully as much as, with our modern methods of rearing premature infants, its chances of survival are relatively great.

Modern opinion is tending toward the acceptance of this view. Lusk protests against postponing resort to the induction of premature labor until the grave symptoms (chiefly cerebral) which precede eclampsia develop. Tarnier, of the French school, holds practically the same opinion. The opponents of this view are certainly many, and their names carry weight; but a careful estimate of the question, both from the stand-point of the woman and of the child, forces on us the conclusion that, dietetic and medicinal measures having failed to ameliorate the symptoms which precede eclampsia, the best interests of both are subserved by the election of premature labor.

Such, briefly outlined, are the indications for the induction of premature labor. In determining the best method for performing the operation, the fact must never be lost sight of that the intent of the operation will ordinarily be to save the woman the greater risk she suffers if allowed to go to term, and also to obtain a living child. To amply satisfy this intent in the individual case, the operation, where election is possible, should be postponed to as near term as is absolutely consistent with the interest of the mother, for thus the chances of the infant's life are increased. Further, the method selected should be one which, while the safest for the woman, takes into full account the phenomena of normal labor, since thus alone are the interests of the child fully subserved. Again, in view of the fact that the child has not attained full maturity, ample preparation should be made beforehand for the rearing of the immature child. Finally, the physician should be prepared to meet every emergency which labor at term might involve; for premature labor may call, before it is completed, for any of the obstetric operations (the forceps, version), and its completion may be followed by the same complications as labor at term (haemorrhage, adherent placenta).

METHODS FOR THE INDUCTION OF PREMATURE LABOR.

Many of the methods which have been proposed for the induction of premature labor are purely of interest from an historical stand-point. Such, for instance, is the administration of medicinal agents,—ergot, rue, quinine, cinnamon, and the like. These drugs will not provoke contractions, although some of them will intensify action when contractions are in force. Again, it has been suggested to start the expulsive action of the uterus by injecting water or air between the membranes and the uterine wall. Such a procedure would doubtless be effective, but should not be countenanced, since it is likely to rupture the membranes, thus imperiling the child, and since it may prove fatal to the woman from the entrance of air into the uterine veins. Vaginal irrigation with hot water is slow and uncertain in action, and, if prolonged, may give rise to local congestion, unfavorable alike to woman and foetus. As will be noted, this method, within limits, is useful as preparatory to other methods, in that by means of it softening of the cervix may be assisted. Electricity is of value only as an adjuvant for hastening labor through re-enforcing contractions when these have once been started. Used alone, this agent is very problematical in effect, and highly uncertain as well.

There are left for consideration the following five methods: 1. Puncture of the membranes. 2 Tamponing the vagina. 3. The injection of glycerin. 4. The insertion of an elastic bougie between the membranes and the uterine wall. 5. Mechanical dilatation of the cervix.

1. *Puncture of the Membranes.*—This may be accomplished in two ways,— by direct puncture through the cervical canal; by insinuating a uterine sound on a sharpened goose-quill between the uterine wall and the membranes and tapping the membranes high up by projecting the quill over the stylet. This method was formerly highly in favor with the Vienna school.

Puncture of the membranes will certainly induce labor, and, where aseptically performed, the method may be ranked as safe for the woman. The method, however, is open to the objection that it does not imitate natural methods, and therefore may imperil the child. In the course of normal labor premature rupture of the membranes invariably leads to tedious labor, and this may entail both maternal and foetal exhaustion. Our aim should be to maintain the dilating water-wedge intact. This is the sound rule of practice in the course of spontaneous labor at term. Similarly, in case of the induction of premature labor, an operation resorted to in the interests of the child as well as in those of the woman, the object should be to maintain the membranes intact, in order to avoid a protracted first stage of labor, with its concomitant risks. Therefore, puncture of the membranes should be dismissed from consideration as a means of inducing premature labor.

2. *Tamponing the Vagina.*—Thorough tamponing of the vagina by means of aseptic tampons will unquestionably, in course of time, provoke uterine contractions, and the more speedily the nearer the woman is to term. The method, if aseptic throughout, carries with it no risk either to the woman or the child, but it is slow in action. Days may elapse before effects on the uterus are noted. Now, when speaking of the indications under which the induction of premature labor was justifiable, we have noted that in pelvic contraction, for instance, it was highly important not to err in the date assigned for the operation, and that under the best possible conditions there existed a chance of error of at least a fortnight. Obviously, no method should be selected for the induction of premature labor which carries with it the strong probability of greatly magnifying this chance of error. The selection of such a method is not fair to the child. Neither under other indications is it fair to the woman. If eclampsia threaten, for instance, and the physician determines that labor should be induced, he cannot afford to place dependence on a method which may not prove effective for days. There exists, indeed, but one indication under which the tampon might till a place, and this is in the event of premature labor being indicated by haemorrhage, due, likely enough, to faulty placental insertion. Here the tampon prevents further haemorrhage whilst the cervix is dilating sufficiently to warrant resort to the next step in treatment. The colpeurynter of the late Karl Braun is an excellent agent for tamponing the vagina in such an instance, but it can never till the place of the aseptic gauze, in private practice certainly, for the reason that it is made of rubber,—an agent which deteriorates with certainty in course of time, and can therefore not be depended upon as to quality. Further, it is not as strictly aseptic as sterilized gauze.

When the tampon is indicated it should be inserted under the strictest asepsis, and with the patient in the knee-chest or in the left lateral position, for thus alone can the vaginal fornices be efficiently packed. An iodoform or boratcd gauze inserted in a continuous strip forms the best tampon. If uterine contractions be not established within thirty hours the strip should be removed, the vagina douched with 2-per-cent. creolin solution or with 1 to 8000 solution of bichloride, and a new strip inserted, unless the cervix is found sufficiently dilated for resort to methods the aim of which is to empty the uterus rapidly.

3. *Injections of Glycerin for the Induction of Prematwe Labor.*—This method has recently been highly commended in Germany, and on the few occasions when it has been tested in this country the success has been fairly uniform. The cases on record are too few to admit of positive statement. In our own hands success has not been marked, but when we tested it the technique had not been perfected as it has at the present. Glycerin, when injected into the uterus between the membranes and the uterine wall, acts by causing exosmosis from the amniotic sac. There is a profuse secretion of fluid from the uterus, and concomitantly uterine contractions set in. The method of procedure is the following:—

The external genitals and the vagina having been rendered thoroughly aseptic, a sterilized gum-elastic catheter is insinuated to the fundus, between the membranes and the uterine wall. The woman is then placed in the knee-chest or in the left lateral position; the catheter is connected by means of a sterilized rubber tube with a glass funnel, and into the funnel is poured sterilized glycerin. Under the influence of gravity this flows into the uterus. The catheter is carefully withdrawn, and the vagina is tamponed with sterilized gauze. The woman should maintain the lateral position for a number of hours, otherwise the glycerin will flow from the uterus and the effects of the injection will be nullified. Uterine contractions should be evoked in the course of a few hours, otherwise the procedure will have to be repeated. Instead of the glass funnel a syringe may be used for injecting the glycerin. It goes without saying that every precaution should be taken against the injection of air into the uterus. The objections to this method which suggest themselves at the present are that it is uncertain in its action, and therefore, where the indication calling for the induction of premature labor is an urgent one, the physician is scarcely justified in taking the chances of failure. A further objection is the risk of rupturing the membranes during the introduction of the catheter,—an accident which, should it occur, places the welfare of the child in an unfavorable light. Further, recent data would seem to prove that nephritis may result. The future, however, may speak with more favor for this method than, at the present, we are inclined to grant it.

4. *The Insertion of an Elastic Bougie between the Membranes and the Uterine Wall Kranse's Method).*—The method of inducing labor by the introduction of an elastic bougie between the membranes and the uterine wall is probably resorted to with greater frequency than any other. The bougie acts as a foreign body, and at a variable interval provokes uterine action with certainty. The method is safe for the woman, provided proper asepsis accompany the insertion of the instrument. There are weighty objections against it, however. In the first place the presence of the bougie in the uterus may not induce labor for some days, and exceptionally not at all, unless it be rotated in the uterus with the aim of separating to a degree the attachment of the membranes. When the induction of premature labor has been duly elected by the physician, nothing is gained by awaiting what in any case may prove the slow action of the bougie; and, for reasons already amply considered, delay may moan the loss of the child. Further, in introducing the bougie (a step not always easy of performance) the membranes may be ruptured, and this accident it is very desirable to avoid in the interest chiefly of the child and partly also of the woman. Rotation of the bougie within the uterus is objectionable: first, on account of the possibility of injuring the placenta, with resulting haemorrhage (perhaps of the concealed type,—so fatal both to the woman and to the child), and, secondly, on account of the risk, again, of rupture of the membranes. Lastly, it is not a very easy matter to asepticize the bougie. Soaking in weak antiseptic solutions will not suffice, and soaking in strong will injure the bougie. The material of which the bougie is constructed forbids its subjection to the most reliable method of obtaining asepsis,—exposure to dry heat. It is evident, therefore, that this method is not an ideal one; still, it is the best at our disposal, and, where the emergency calling for the induction of premature labor was not a very urgent one, this method has answered well. In case of urgency, however, it must be supplemented by a further step, which we will shortly describe. *Technique of Krause's Method.*—The instruments requisite are a speculum (preferably the Sims), a steel-branched dilator, and a tenaculum. The external genitals and the vagina having been thoroughly asepticized, the woman is placed in the left lateral position, and the cervix is exposed through the speculum. The tenaculum is inserted into the anterior lip of the cervix to steady the uterus, and the cervical canal is dilated to the extent of a half-inch by the steel-branched dilator. This step is requisite in order to enable the passage of the bougie with least risk of injuring the integrity of the membranes. The asepticized bougie is then carefully insinuated to the fundus, between the membranes and the uterine wall. A tampon of sterilized gauze is inserted into the vagina to keep the bougie from slipping from the uterus. The woman is put to bed and remains there until uterine contractions are evoked. In the event of these contractions not supervening within twenty-four hours, the bougie must be removed, the vagina douched with creolin solution, and, if the emergency is still not pressing, a second sterilized bougie is inserted. If uterine contractions have been evoked, then, if the

emergency be not pressing, the progress of labor is left to nature. In the event of a complication arising calling for speedy delivery, the physician may resort to the method shortly to be described. 5. *Dilatation of the Cervix as a Means of Inducing Premature Labor.*—With this method as a working basis, labor may be induced and completed within fairly normal limits, with less risk to the woman and the child than by any other method. Under this heading, then, the operation for the induction of premature labor will be described.

The operation having been elected, ever—except in strict emergency—under the support of a consultant, the physician will ordinarily have ample time to thoroughly cleanse the intestinal canal by the administration of one or another laxative, or, failing sufficient time for this, the lower bowel, at any rate, should be emptied by a copious enema. Convalescence from any obstetrical operation is favored when the great emunctory of the system is neither clogged nor torpid. The bladder is emptied and the field of operation is carefully asepticized as follows: The labia and vestibule are thoroughly washed with soap and water, and then with a 2-per-cent. creolin or with a 1 to 5000 sublimate solution. By means of a small tooth-brush the vagina is similarly prepared. Simple douching of the vagina is not sufficient, since the folds of the canal cannot thus be rendered aseptic. The physician, and whoever assists him, should scrub his hands with soap and water, and next immerse them in a 2-per-cent. creolin or in a 1 to 2000 sublimate solution.

The instruments necessary are the following: A Sims speculum, an intrauterine forceps, a tenaculum, a steel-branched dilator. These are to be carefully disinfected beforehand, and at the time of use may be placed in sterilized water or in an antiseptic solution, according to the preference of the individual operator. About two yards of sterilized gauze, two inches in width, are also needed.

Such are the precautions which are strictly essential in order to guard the woman against her main risk,—septic infection. The bladder having been emptied, the woman is placed in the left lateral position, the speculum inserted, and the tenaculum fixed in the anterior cervical lip. In rare instances it may be necessary to dilate the cervical canal to the extent of half an inch before proceeding to the next step; this, however, will prove the exception beyond the seven and one-half months of gestation, owing to the softened condition of the cervical tissues at this period. The sterilized gauze is grasped by the packing forceps and carried into the cervix up to and not beyond the internal os. The cervical canal is thus progressively packed full, and the remainder of the gauze is utilized to tampon the upper vagina. The object of the gauze is twofold; it will in all probability excite uterine contractions, but, if it do not, it mechanically dilates the cervix to a sufficient degree to enable the next step to be resorted to. The patient is placed in bed, and, in the event of the presence of the gauze being painful, a suppository of two grains of codeine may be inserted into the rectum. Within ten to twenty-four hours the gauze will probably excite contractions, with the greater certainty the nearer the woman is to term. The physician's duty now becomes expectant or active, according to the emergency which has demanded the induction of premature labor. In the event of the indication for rapidly terminating labor not being urgent, the gauze is removed, under aseptic precautions, and the labor may be allowed to progress toward its natural termination. The physician's duty is purely passive, even as it is during the progress of normal labor. This applies particularly to instances where labor is induced in the presence of a contracted pelvis, where the lapse of even twenty-four hours has no untoward effect on either the woman or the child. Here, until full dilatation of the cervix, artificial aid is only called for under stringent indication from the side of the woman or the child, such as haemorrhage or evidence of foetal heart-failure. It is absolutely essential to maintain the integrity of the membranes, since the cervix once dilated, the safety of the woman or of the child, or the degree of pelvic contraction may call for the deliberate election of version.

In the event of contractions not having been induced, if no emergency requiring specially active measures be present, the physician, under strict asepsis, may insert another strip of gauze; but if the indications be pressing, the cervical tissues have been dilated to a degree by the gauze, and have been softened so that it is possible to resort to the next step in the operation, which, in the vast majority of cases, will give the physician full control of the case.

The aim of the step to which we now pass is to secure full dilatation of the cervix or, in any event, sufficient dilatation to enable the physician to resort to version, the conditions under the premises being still favorable for this operation. According to whether the indication for interference be urgent or not, the physician may elect one of two procedures,—the first, in case delay of a few hours seems allowable; the second, if delivery is necessary within as brief a space of time as is consistent with inflicting no damage on the cervix and lower uterine segment. Both measures entail mechanical dilatation of the cervix.

The first method consists in the use of Barnes's hydrostatic bags or their essential modification, McLean's bags; the second depends on the use of the hand, a method not highly favored because of the objectionable and erroneous term applied to it,— *accouchement force.*

The difference between Barnes's and McLean's bags is that the former has but one compartment, removal being necessitated for the insertion of progressively larger sizes. McLean's bag, on the other hand, has two compartments, so that when the cervical canal has been dilated to the full extent of one compartment the other may be brought into action without removal of the bag.

The method of using these hydrostatic dilators is the following: The vagina and the external genitals having been asepticized, and the bag and the forceps having been similarly treated, the bag is seized in the grasp of the forceps, and, under the guidance of one or two fingers in the vagina, it is inserted into the cervical canal just beyond the internal os. If uterine contractions are present the attempt at insertion should be made in the interval of the contractions, in order to avoid possible rupture of the membranes. The bag being in place, the forceps is withdrawn, the rubber tube of the bag is connected with a Davidson syringe, and the bag is distended with sterilized water. The object in using sterilized water is to avoid septicizing the uterus, in case the bag should rupture. The rubber tube is then clamped and the patient is put to bed. Ordinarily, after the lapse of two hours, the cervical canal has been dilated to the full extent of the single compartment of the McLean bag, and the tube of the second compartment is connected with the syringe and similarly distended with sterilized water. In about an hour more the cervix has been sufficiently dilated to enable the physician to resort to delivery of the fœtus, preferably by version, if the integrity of the membranes has been maintained.

It is at once obvious that this method will not answer where the emergency requiring interference is urgent, as, for instance, in case of placenta praevia or eclampsia. Here time is an important factor, and a more rapid method is called for. Of late years a method of rapid dilatation, called by the French the *accouchement force,* has been resuscitated from unmerited oblivion, and in the presence of the emergencies just noted it offers the best aid to the woman, and also about the only hope for the child. The reason why the method fell into disuse and has been reprobated by obstetricians generally up to a comparatively recent date is because of the name which was applied to it. The fact is that absolutely no force need be used or is used in securing dilatation. The method depends for its success on the well-recognized fact that any muscle in the body will yield to continuously applied pressure. The procedure is, of course, tiresome to the operator, but the clinical results which may be secured through timely resort to it will amply compensate. The technique is the following: The woman being deeply anaesthetized, and the genital tract having been thoroughly asepticized, the hand is introduced into the vagina and the index finger is inserted into the cervical canal. Steady pressure is maintained, and shortly it will be found possible to insert the middle finger. Progressively thus finger after finger is inserted, until the entire hand has been introduced. The fist is then doubled and in a few minutes the remaining obstacle to dilatation will be found to yield and the physician can at once take the subsequent steps requisite for delivery.

We would again impress the fact that this method should be reserved for strict emergency. The risk the method subjects the woman to is laceration of the cervix, the rent from which might even extend into the lower uterine segment. This major accident should not, however, occur unless the cardinal rule is neglected, which is to use absolutely no force, but to cause the cervix to yield to the applied pressure. In the event of a minor laceration of the cervix occurring, the immediate operation on the cervix should be performed. This will be described in its proper place.

Both these methods—the use of the hydrostatic dilators as well as manual dilatation—evoke uterine contractions as well as dilate the cervical canal. These methods constitute at the present the ideal ones of inducing labor. They fulfill every requisite indication. They are aseptic. They start labor by the natural method, by evoking uterine contractions without the possible sacrifice of the child through premature rupture of the membranes; as a rule, they enable delivery to be effected within fairly normal limits. They necessitate, of course, the constant attention of the physician after the completion of the first step, the provoking of uterine contractions, but, as noted under indications, such attendance is requisite in order to fulfill strictly the aim of the operation, which is the safety both of the woman and the child. At any time it may become necessary to interfere actively in the interests of either. The first stage once completed, labor is ended spontaneously or by forceps or version, according to the individual case.

Prognosis.—The prognosis of the operation for the induction of premature labor obviously will vary according to the indication which requires it. If resorted to in the presence of eclampsia or placenta praevia, the result both for woman and child is necessarily more unfavorable than when, the emergency not being an extreme one, the physician has time at his disposal for the due election of each and every step. Everything, further, it should be re-iterated, depends on the careful observance of strict asepsis. Whilst the prognosis should be guarded, in general it may be stilted that the operation should not have a mortality rate. Election of the operation and asepsis are the key-notes of success.

As regards the child, its chances of survival are the less the earlier the stage of gestation at which the operation is resorted to. Under the thirty-sixth week the infant can only be reared through the exercise of every possible care. In hospital practice, with modern appliances, it ought to be possible to save, at the thirty-sixth week (the ninth lunar month), fully 85 per cent, of the children. This has been accomplished by means of the incubator and forced feeding. At the Paris Maternity, 30 per cent, of children at the sixth month have been thus reared, 63.6 per cent, at seven months, and 85.7 per cent, at eight months. These figures refer to calendar months. In private practice, and particularly in country districts, it is not possible to always obtain an incubator, and the physician must do the best possible by means of an improvised incubator, such as an oven, the temperature being maintained at about 90 F. Recently, an inexpensive and portable incubator, so simple in construction that trained intellect is not necessary for its management, has been devised by Marx, of New York, and the hope is that before long every physician who contemplates the induction of premature labor will take steps to secure one in advance.

This incubator consists of a box made of well-seasoned hard wood, 21 inches long, 20 inches wide, and 14.4 inches high, lined throughout with sheet zinc, between which and the wood is a layer of sheet asbestos. It is divided by a partition into two unequal portions, one of which, slightly wider than the other, is the incubator proper, the other containing the heatgenerating apparatus. This latter is a copper boiler of the capacity of one quart, resting on a tripod, underneath which is a Bunsen burner or an alcohol-lamp, which supplies heat to the water. Passing from the boiler through the partition and winding about the coils over the V-bottom of the incubator portion is a -inch pipe about 10 feet in length, terminating in a free vent outside the box. The steam thus received in a suitable vessel, condenses and gives us an index of the condition of the boiler. The top of the boiler projects through the box and is closed by a metal cap, which unscrews so that the V-boiler may be readily replenished with water. In the incubator proper there is a well-padded basket suspended so that its bottom is about 5 inches above the coil of the steam-pipe. A glass plate sliding in grooves acts as a cover, which may be partially or entirely withdrawn to aid in the ventilation, which is supplied by numerous holes drilled in the walls of the box. A thermometer is fastened horizontally to the top of the basket, immediately beneath the glass slide.

This simple apparatus commends itself on account of its relative cheapness, thus bringing it within the reach of even people of moderate means in whose families the operation of the induction of premature labor becomes an operation of election. Even so, we question whether, outside of maternity hospitals and the homes of the well-to-do, it will often be practicable to rear infants under the thirty-second week of gestation, in view of the necessity of having an attendant to watch the incubator night and day.

CHAPTER III FORCEPS.

It is not intended here to enter into the history of the subject at all, nor to describe the various instruments and their modifications which are in general use. The special modification of the instrument is of very much less service than an accurate knowledge of the use of the instrument. Recognizing the fact that traction is the essential power of forceps, it will appear that any instrument which is easily kept clean, easily adjusted to the child's head, and which is rigid enough to pre vent slipping, will be the instrument which will meet the greatest number of requirements.

Numbers of instruments have been devised, which, though not perfect, will so nearly meet these requirements as to leave little to be desired. A forceps which is in very general use, and which is capable of being adapted to a large number of cases, is Elliott's (Fig. 32). This is a long, well-curved, and somewhat heavy instrument, which has an adjustable screw in the handle, by means of which the amount of pressure on the head can be regulated. While this is a convenience, it is no easy matter to keep the screw aseptic, and the same end may be gained by placing a folded towel between the handles of instruments not furnished with this attachment.

An instrument which is not in very general use, but which undoubtedly possesses merit, is known as Hunter's (Fig. 33). This instrument, having almost no handle, is grasped by means of a bar formed by the locking of the two blades. A firm purchase is attained in tins way, and the hand is so near the head of the child that but little leverage force is possible. The shortness of the handles renders this forceps easy of application.

In addition to possessing some instrument which will meet the requirements mentioned, the operator who wishes to be prepared to meet emergencies must, of necessity, supply himself with some instrument which will permit him to make use of the principle of axis-traction. This can be found best perhaps in the instrument as devised by Tarnier and modified by Lusk (Fig. 34). The disadvantages of this instrument are that it is heavy and adds an amount of weight to the obstetric bag which is objectionable. It is somewhat expensive, thus deterring some from supplying themselves with it. The axis-traction rods which have been devised by Reynolds (Fig. 36) possess the advantages of being light, taking up but little room, and are comparatively inexpensive. They may be attached to any pair of fenestrated forceps. This contrivance consists of a pair of steel rods, which terminate at their upper ends in flat buttons intended to engage in the lower extremity of the fenestra; and at their lower ends in hooks, which are received by rings connected with a transverse traction handle. The appliance is perfectly simple, and any operator can easily apply it to his ordinary forceps. They may be fastened to the forceps-blades either before or after the blades have been adjusted to the child's head.

Traction is not the only force of which the forceps is capable, for compression and leverage are coincident to a greater or less degree.

In order that the forceps may not slip, a certain amount of compression is necessary when traction is being made. It is wise to remember this specially in those cases where the operation is prolonged, in order that injury may not result to the child. From time to time the instrument should be unlocked and the handles slightly separated, thus liberating the foetal head. The forceps is not used for this compression force; it is simply an unfortunate condition, without which traction cannot be made. It is better that traction should be of an intermittent character, if for no other reason than that the head may be relieved of this necessary compression at least every two minutes. Most authors hold that any form of leverage to be obtained by forceps is not only objectionable, but absolutely harmful. The use of the swinging or pendulum motion during traction may easily result in dangerous consequences to the mother, and should not be attempted. Without any doubt, a very slight up-and-down motion will facilitate the extraction; but it must be borne in mind that, at the same time, the free ends of the forceps may be plowing into the maternal soft parts.

Direct traction is fraught with so little danger to the mother, and will so certainly be successful in those cases where the forceps is indicated, that it would be better never to resort to this pendulum motion. Instrumental rotation should not be attempted, for maternal injury is almost certain to result. However, it is necessary for the physician to bear in mind that if the forceps has been applied before rotation has taken place he must be careful not to prevent it by rigidly holding his instrument.

Indications.—It would be almost impossible to mention all the indications for the application of the forceps. In a general way it may be said that inability of the mother's expulsive forces to overcome the obstacles to delivery is one of the most frequent indications.

Secondly, any cause which requires that the delivery should be accomplished rapidly, either in the interest of the mother or the child, provided, for other reasons, that the forceps is not contra-indicated, makes its application justifiable.

Forceps should not be applied to the hydrocephalic head, a decomposing foetus, nor upon a perforated head. If applied to the hydrocephalic head or one that is decomposing, it will almost certainly fail to hold, and, even if successful, the end gained is not commensurate with the risk of injury to the mother. The perforated head can be better handled with a cephalotribe.

Forceps should not be applied until the os is three-quarters dilated or dilatable, nor until the membranes have ruptured and retracted. If the membranes have not retracted, there is the possibility that they may be grasped by the forceps and placental detachment occur.

The actual size of the os is of less importance than its dilatability. Forceps should not be applied until the elasticity of the cervix justifies the easy introduction of the blades.

There must be no mechanical obstruction on the part of the pelvic canal which will prevent the delivery of the child without unusual force. Carcinoma of the cervix, inasmuch as the cervix is rendered so pliable, is a contra-indication to the application of forceps.

Forceps should not be applied where the foetal head and the pelvic canal are so disproportionate that the probability of delivering a live child seems small.

Finally, forceps should not be applied until the head has engaged.

In regard to the time which should be allowed to elapse before the obstetrician resorts to instrumental delivery, it must be remembered that it is a question of conditions, and not minutes or hours. Undoubtedly many women would escape that condition of pelvic relaxation, which is so often seen, following tardy deliveries, if forceps were used before the muscles entering into the pelvic floor were paralyzed from overstretching. As soon as it is evident that the *vis a tergo* is not sufficient to overcome the resistance, then forceps should be applied. Another very safe rule to remember is: whenever the head fails to recede after a contraction of the uterus, forceps should be applied. The failure of the head to recede after a contraction shows that undue pressure is being made on the soft parts of the pelvic canal.

Anaesthesia.—Although it is probable that the extraction of the child with forceps is but slightly more painful than normal delivery, yet it is rarely justifiable to apply forceps until the patient is thoroughly under the influence of the anaesthetic. The danger which may result from some sudden motion on the part of the woman is greater than the danger of the aiuesthctic, to say nothing of the increased ease of extraction on the part of the obstetrician. Chloroform is so much more rapid in its effects, and leaves so little to be desired as an anaesthetic, that it is preferable to ether. The patient should be anaesthetized to the surgical degree before the instrument is applied.

Many authors hold that the application of forceps is only justifiable in head presentations. Undoubtedly it will seldom be necessary to apply it to the breech, but there are conditions which will render the application of forceps to the full breech very advantageous.

It is absolutely necessary to make a correct diagnosis of the position of the child and the causation of the tardy natural delivery before the application of forceps. Before the examination is made which is to determine these points, it is better that the obstetrician have everything in readiness, so that no delay may occur. lie should see that the usual heart stimulants are at hand. An hypodermatic syringe and fluid extract of ergot, together with other oxytocics, should be in readiness. The instrument should be sterilized and placed in a basin containing 1 to 100 creolin solution.

Inasmuch as in forceps cases repeated digital examinations are made, it is wise to exercise unusual care in rendering the hands aseptic. They should be thoroughly scrubbed with soap and hot water, and afterward *immersed* in 1 to 1000 bichloride-of-mercury solution for five minutes. The patient should be anaesthetized and turned across the bed so that the hips will extend well over its edge; the knees can be held by two assistants sitting on either side of the patient. The anaesthetic should be given into the hands of a physician who will have no other duty to attend to.

The external genitals and vagina should be cleansed with soap and water and a soft scrubbing-brush, and afterward douched either with 1 to 3000 bichloride-of-mercury solution or 1 to 100 creolin solution.

After palpating the abdomen one hand should be passed into the vagina if the head is high, and with two fingers the operator should carefully palpate the fontanelles. If there be any doubt about their relation to the pelvic canal he should seek an car, and finding it will enable the diagnosis to be made certainly. At the same time he can determine if any obstruction on the part of the mother exists. The foetal heart-sounds should be listened to, for their character will enable him to determine somewhat the effects of tardy delivery on the life of the child. The forceps is usually applied while the patient is on her back, though some prefer the left lateral posture. The bladder and rectum should be emptied before any operative procedure is undertaken.

The operator, having assured himself of the exact position of the child's head, and that there are no contra-indications to delivery by the forceps, proceeds to apply it.

The blades, for purposes of designation, are known as right and left, corresponding to the right and left sides of the pelvic canal. The left blade should be introduced first on account of the method of locking. The left blade, grasped near the handle with the left hand, is introduced into the vagina (Plate IV and Fig. 37). Two or more fingers of the right hand passed into the vagina until the head is felt will serve as a guide to its

Fig. 37.—Introduction of the Let t lilade of the Forceps.

introduction. The blade is made to glide along the palmar surface of the right hand and pass between the fingers of that hand and the head. It is necessary to remember the two curves of the forceps in introducing it. As the blade passes the fingers the handle is to be depressed and carried slightly outward. At no time must force be used in its introduction. If the blade cannot be made to easily adjust itself, it is better to withdraw it entirely and make another attempt. Force is so certain to do injury to the soft parts that it is never justifiable. After the left blade has been introduced its handle should be given into the hands of an assistant, and the right blade introduced. Here the left hand acts as the guide and the right hand manages the blade (Fig. 38). No attempt should be made to introduce the blades during a contraction of the uterus.

It is customary to apply the blades first to the sides of the pelvis, irrespective of the position of the child's head, and afterward, if possible, have them grasp the child's head in its biparietal diameter. As soon as the blades are passed and adjusted, they should be locked (Fig. 39). This is usually accomplished easily by slightly depressing both handles. Should

Fig. 38.—The Left Blade Introduced; the Right Blade (in Outline) Ready to bo Introduced.

this not accomplish the desired end they may be advanced or slightly withdrawn, and another attempt made to lock them. Forced locking must not be attempted. The very fact that the blades will not easily lock indicates that there is either faulty application or else the case is not one in which forceps should be used.

There is no operation which calls for more gentleness, judgment, and patience than the application of forceps. It is always necessary to bear in mind the possibility of including the mother's soft parts in the grasp of the forceps, and the injury which would result therefrom.

It is necessary to study the subject of forceps operations in their various phases, inasmuch as they each present their own peculiarities.

The operations may be divided into low, medium, and high applications. Again, whether the occiput is anterior or posterior, and whether the head is proportionate to the pelvic canal or not.

The Application of Low Forceps, Occipitoanterior Position,

Fig. 39.—The Forceps Adjusted and Ready to be Locked.

Head and Birth-Canal Proportionate. —This operation is the most simple of all forceps deliveries. It is indicated when for any reason it is an advantage to mother or child that the labor be terminated. These are the cases where non-interference so often results in injury to the mother's pelvic floor, the head remaining on the pelvic floor for so long a time that the levator ani muscle and the triangular ligaments are not able to regain their tonicity after the labor and their diaphragmatic action is impaired.

It must be borne in mind that the abdominal muscles play by far the greater part in the act of expelling the head from the vulva, and in women of poor muscular development or in those who have become thoroughly exhausted from a prolonged first stage the muscular force necessary to expel the head may be wanting. Many of these women would undoubtedly deliver themselves if left alone; but the question arises whether or not they will not suffer more injury, and of a more permanent character, if unaided, than could possibly result from the application of low forceps. It is not intended by this to mean that every woman should be delivered with forceps as soon as the head is low down, but simply as an opinion that many women are permanently injured by reason of an unnecessarily prolonged second stage.

Under strict aseptic precautions, as already mentioned, the blades are applied over the biparietal diameter of the child's head. As soon as locking has been accomplished, it is well to make tentative traction to see that they have a firm grasp.

The instrument should be grasped with the right hand, with palmar surface downward. Should the instrument have transverse shoulders, the index and middle fingers should be placed over one shoulder and the remaining fingers over the other. In using Hunter's forceps it is often a relief to place a towel over the cross-bar and with the right hand grasp the towel. (Plate V, Fig. 1.) The left hand should be placed against the patient's buttocks, with one finger over the fourchette. This will enable the operator to determine just how much force he is exerting on the perineum. Traction should be made downward, or as nearly so as the perineum will permit, thus accentuating flexion (Fig. 40). Pendulum or swinging force during traction is contra-indicated. Firm traction exerted for not more than one minute will accomplish the extraction if persisted in. It should be the operator's attempt to imitate nature as nearly as possible in preparing the perineum for the delivery of the head. This can be done by allowing the head to recede after each traction. He should also release the grasp of the forceps slightly at each recession, that the child may not be injured.

In the majority of cases calling for instrumental extraction pains are so infrequent that it is not wise for the operator to wait for the help which uterine contractions may give him, but he should make traction irrespective of their presence. Welldirected abdominal pressure on the part of an assistant will be of undoubted value. If it is evident that perineal laceration is impending, it is better to at once perform episiotomy. This little operation is no doubt worthy of more consideration than it has ever-received. The measure is a simple one, consisting only in relieving the strain on the perineum by making a lateral incision on either side of the vulvar orifice. (Plate V, Fig. 2.) The incision need not be more than an eighth of an inch in depth and half an inch long, extending up into the vagina. It is not likely that haemorrhage of any consequence will result from this procedure, but, even if it should, a continuous catgut stitch will control it without difficulty.

As soon as the occiput is brought well down underneath the pubic arch, the forceps should be removed and the head delivered *between* pains, by introducing the finger into the rectum and, finding the chin, tilting it out over the perineum. As soon as the head is delivered it should be held so that the shoulders may not be driven through the vulvar outlet during a pain; but as soon as the contraction, which is nearly always excited by the delivery of the head, has subsided, they may be lifted out as was the head.

Low Forceps in Occipito-poaterior Position, with Partial J Potation.—It has been shown that firm uterine contractions, forcing the foetus to travel over the inclined planes of the pelvis and resisted by a firm perineum, will cause the occiput to rotate forward. Should any of these factors be absent rotation may not be complete, and the fœtus will occupy an oblique position with occiput posterior. Usually, by giving the mother a rest, firm contractions will ensue and anterior rotation and normal delivery take place. It often happens, however, that in the interest of mother or child instrumental delivery becomes necessary. After a very careful examination, so that the exact position of the occiput is made out, forceps should be applied in one of two ways: either directly to the sides of the pelvis or else in an oblique position.

The latter is more difficult, but is preferable on account of the lessened risks to the child. The forceps should be applied in that oblique diameter which is not occupied by the head. This will cause the blades to grasp the biparietal diameter of the head. The rule that the left blade should be introduced first should be disregarded here, unless it be at the same time the anterior blade, for tins is the difficult one and should be first introduced. Unusual care must be taken to guard the mother's soft parts from injury. The forceps should be unlocked after each traction, which not only lessens the danger to the child, but also by releasing the head permits rotation to take place. At no time must instrumental rotation be attempted, nor, on the other hand, must natural rotation be prevented. Oftentimes it is wise to remove the forceps altogether and readjust it over the biparietal diameter, which may have changed its position. By patience and absence of any desire on the part of th» operator to hasten the rotation, the head will often gradually mold itself, and under the tractions of the forceps, which acts as a re-inforcement to the expellant forces, rotate anteriorly.

If, after patient and gentle efforts, it be impossible to adjust the forceps over the biparietal diameter, it should be applied directly to the sides of the pelvis. The same care must be exercised here that the mother's soft tissues are not injured. It is also imperative that tractions should not be prolonged longer than a minute, and that the grasp of the forceps be relaxed between tractions. The child is put to such a disadvantage, even under these circumstances, that its life is often seriously jeopardized and the operation is done primarily in the interest of the mother.

Low Forceps in Occipito-posterior Position.—It is the general opinion among obstetricians that few abnormalities produce 4 a more difficult condition to terminate successfully than those cases where the occiput has rotated posteriorly and is wedged in the hollow of the sacrum. Fortunately they are not very frequent, for the child's condition is most perilous and injury to the mother's soft parts almost certain.

It is far better to delay the application of forceps in these cases as long as possible, that, under continued uterine contractions, anterior rotation may occur. If, however, the mother is showing signs of exhaustion, or if the foctal heart become feeble, then there is no other resort but to apply forceps. Delay beyond this point is not admissible.

The patient should be anaesthetized and the parts rendered aseptic, as before suggested. Carefully guarding the soft parts, the blades are applied to either side of the child's head. A moderate amount of pressure is necessary to prevent the blades slipping, but by relaxing the grasp frequently the injury to the child will be greatly lessened. As soon as the forehead is made to appear beneath the pubic arch it is well to remove the forceps, and, unless the reasons for immediate extraction are urgent, it is well to give nature a chance to rotate the occiput anteriorly. Otherwise, in place of making traction horizontally, as is necessary when bringing the forehead underneath the pubic arch, the handles should be lowered as far as the perineum will permit. This manoeuvre will cause marked extension of the head and the forehead will be brought underneath the pubic rami. Forced extension now will cause the forehead to clear the pubes. The forceps should now be removed and, passing two fingers into the rectum, the head should be flexed until the occiput escapes over the perineum.

Laceration of the perineum will be almost certain to occur, and it should be repaired at once.

Fig. 41.—Showing Direction of Traction in Face Presentation.

As already stated, these cases are among the most difficult ones found in obstetrics, and one of the hardest things to resist is the desire to attempt instrumental rotation. It will only be necessary to remember to what unusual risks this will subject the mother, to deter one from this procedure.

Low Forceps in Face Presentations.—The application of forceps in face presentations, when that condition has not been diagnosed until after the face is well down in the pelvic canal, should be delayed as long as is consistent with the safety of mother and child, in order that anterior rotation of the chin may occur. This rotation is nearly always tardy, and sometimes does not take place at all. Manual rotation of the head, if not too firmly wedged, is permissible and sometimes successful, but at no time should forceps be used to bring about this rotation. If the chin has rotated anteriorly, forceps should be applied directly to the sides of the child's head. A firm grasp must be taken and some compression used to prevent the blades slipping. Traction should be made horizontally until the chin is brought underneath the pubic arch, when the handles should be raised and the cranial vault and occiput lifted over the perineum. If the chin is turned posteriorly and the head is wedged in the pelvic outlet, there is so little probability that a living child can be extracted that it seems to be the part of conservative treatment to turn the attention entirely to the welfare of the mother and do craniotomy, or, in favorable cases, symphysiotomy. *Forceps in Breech Presentations.*—Forceps should not be applied to the breech until after it has firmly engaged. When, however, the breech has entered the pelvic canal, and yet is too high to permit the finger passing over the groin or the application of the fillet, Tarnier's axis-traction forceps will be most advantageous. A dilated or dilatable os will render the operation so much more easy of success that this should be accomplished before the application of forceps. The majority of these cases are met in old primiparae, where the parts are more than usually rigid, and the time spent in dilating the cervix will not be wasted. If rotation has occurred, the blades should be applied over the sacrum and posterior aspect of the thigh.

It is here that caution will be necessary to prevent the blades impinging so firmly on the parts that the child will be injured, and at the same time firmly enough so that they will not slip and injure the mother's soft parts. Hence it is better to make tentative traction at first, to see that the grasp is firm. The application of the principle of axis-traction to forceps enables the operator to use very much less force in the extraction, inasmuch as the resistance caused by the pressure of the presenting part against the anterior pelvic wall is very much lessened. Traction should be made only during a contraction of the uterus, unless the pains be too infrequent. If this should be the case, it is better to imitate the methods of nature and permit the recession of the breech after each traction. The rigidity of the canal will rapidly lessen under the influence of the advance of the breech, and the integrity of the soft parts will more likely be preserved.

If this intermittent traction is used, a very small amount of force will accomplish the delivery of the breech. Should the hips be transverse, it is better to attempt manual rotation first. If this is not possible, then the blades should be applied to the lateral surfaces of the thighs (Fig. 42). It is not expedient to allow the blades to embrace the crests of the ilia, inasmuch as the bones are too compressible and the forceps is almost certain to slip. In all cases well-directed pressure over the fundus will greatly facilitate the extraction.

The Application of Medium Forceps.—Most authors refer to all forceps operations above the inferior strait as high forceps, and confuse in this way two very different operations. When the head has firmly engaged, indicating that its greatest diameter has entered the pelvic inlet, it seems better to consider it as being in a medium position, and, should it become arrested there and necessitate extraction, to call the operation medium forceps. This condition depends either on the disproportion of the head and the birth-canal or on lack of uterine force to overcome the resistance which is normally present.

This operation is fraught with far more danger than low forceps, for the blades of the instrument must of necessity enter the lower uterine segment, when the most extreme caution will be necessary to prevent injury to the uterus. Hence it is advisable to delay the application of forceps until instrumental delivery seems imperative to the mother or child, or both. If the undilated cervix is preventing the advancement of the head, it is far better to *manually* dilate it than to use the forceps as a dilating force, as is advised by many. Should cicatrization from any cause render the cervical tissue non-dilatable, the little procedure of nicking the cervical ring, as will be described in the chapter on "Version," will greatly facilitate the dilatation. In a recent case, where there was a distinct history of diphtheritic vaginitis in early childhood, one of the authors encountered this condition very markedly pronounced. The head was firmly engaged and it was with difficulty that one finger could be introduced into the os, although the woman had been in labor twenty-four hours.

After making five or six shallow cuts through this hardened ring, manual dilatation was completed in eleven minutes. This procedure is fraught with no danger to the child and less to the mother than when dilatation is accomplished by alternately drawing the head down and allowing it to recede. If the delay in advancement is due to lack of uterine force, this organ will often resume its energy if the patient is given a small dose of quinine,—5 to 10 grains. Should it become necessary, however, to apply forceps, the most strict aseptic precautions will be necessary. The patient should be completely anaesthetized and prepared, as has already been stated. The operator should be certain that the blades do not embrace any of the cervical tissue in their grasp. This can be prevented by recognizing the exact relation of the cervix to the child's head, and permitting the blade to enter the lower uterine segment between the fingers and the foetal head.

Medium forceps is usually applied directly to the sides of the pelvis (Fig. 44). Axis-traction forceps in these cases can certainly accomplish more with less force than any other instrument. Although, in the majority of cases, when the forceps is thus applied, it will be found that the blades have grasped the head in its oblique diameter, yet if the grasp of the forceps is frequently relaxed the injury to the child will not be great. As the head advances under the influence of axis-traction anterior rotation will probably occur, and the free mobility, which is insured by the handle of the traction rod, will permit this rotation more certainly than if the ordinary long forceps is used.

As soon as the head has been brought down to the floor of the pelvis, it is better to remove the axis-traction instrument, and, if it is necessary to extract, complete the operation with the ordinary forceps. If the axis-traction forceps be not at hand, and the ordinary forceps be used, the operator must make traction as nearly downward as the perineum will permit, bearing in mind at the same time that the pelvic curve of the blades may be making undue pressure against the anterior aspect of the uterus. At the same time, if the handles are raised the presenting part will simply be forced against the symphysis and further advancement be prevented. Hence it will be necessary to exercise unusual patience, and at no time attempt to dislodge the head by the application of brute force.

High Forceps.—It has already been stated that while the head is movable above the brim forceps should not be applied.

In rare cases where the waters have drained away and the uterus has firmly contracted around the fœtus, rendering version impossible, simply as a tentative measure forceps may be applied.

It is needless to say that the Aery greatest care must be taken, or else serious if not fatal injury to the mother will result. The patient should be thoroughly anaesthetized and the entire hand gently introduced into the vagina. It must be remembered that after uterine retraction has taken place the possibility of rupture is increased and no harsh measures must be adopted. It should be the aim of the obstetrician to determine, if possible, the cause of the failure of the head to engage. If it is due to contraction of the pelvis to any marked extent, it will be useless to attempt to drag the head into and through the pelvic canal. If the true conjugate is less than three and three-fourths inches, with a normally-developed foetus at full term, forceps should not be used.

If u¡)on examination the pelvic canal be normal, and it is found that early loss of waters has taken place and that uterine contractions have not been of normal force, then the forceps may be applied while the head is still above the brim if version be contra-indicated. As in medium forceps, the cervix must be dilated before the forceps is applied. Carefully guarding the blade with the right hand, the left blade should be introduced. No force must be used, and if the blades cannot be adjusted to the sides of the pelvis without force the operation should be discontinued. If, however, they can be applied, only gentle force must be used to see if the head can be made to engage. Axis-traction forceps should be used. Should the head engage, the after-conduction of the case will be the same as in medium forceps.

Prognosis.—The application of low forceps should be attended with absolutely no mortality to either mother or child. When the head has firmly engaged, yet has not descended into the pelvis, forceps, when applied under the rules of asepsis already given, should not be attended by a mortality to the mother, and, where there is no malposition or disproportion, should be alike safe to the child.

In the high operation, where the head is yet above the brim, the prognosis for both mother and child is very much less satisfactory. Extensive laceration of the soft parts and even rupture of the uterus may occur. Experienced operators hesitate before applying high forceps, realizing the great risk to the patient. The outlook for the child, on account of the prolonged compression of the head, is even more serious. Although the frequent unlocking of the blades will afford a greater degree of safety to the child, its life not only is often jeopardized, but injury to the cranium may result in fatal convulsions or epilepsy.

CHAPTER IV. VERSION.

The term "version" applies to all operative methods for changing the relation between the long axis of the child and the long axis of the uterus.

Inasmuch as version is but another expression for turning, it also embraces the operation for converting an occipito-posterior position into an anterior one while the child is *in ufero,* even though the long axes of the child and the uterus remain unchanged. By means of this operative interference the cephalic or pelvic pole may be caused to present. The breech may be changed for the head, the head for the breech, or a transverse either to the breech or head.

Again, as is stated above, the back of the child may be turned toward the abdomen of the mother. Before any operative procedure is performed it is absolutely necessary to determine the exact relationship which the child bears to the uterus; also the mechanical obstruction which is to be overcome, and an estimate of the comparative size of the child's head and the pelvic outlet.

Ordinarily this can be determined by abdominal palpation and vaginal examination, both of which methods should be resorted to. External palpation is a procedure too seldom used, and those who will accustom themselves to study every obstetrical case in this way will be surprised to see how soon experience will yield happy results. It is so very important to know just what position the child is in, that if, as is sometimes the case, it is impossible to gain the proper information from these two methods of examination, it is better to introduce the hand into the vagina and one or two fingers through the os. In this way a positive diagnosis can be made. At the same time other valuable information can be gained, viz., the absence or character of the pulsation of the cord; the low implantation of the placenta, if such be the case; the normal or otherwise prominence of the sacral arch, and, in cases of slightly deformed pelves, whether or not one or both of the pubic rami encroach on the pelvic outlet. It is necessary to determine as nearly as possible all these, conditions, or else there will be far too many cases of perforation of the after-coming head, with the too late realization that the case was not one on which version should have been performed.

The multiplication of terms is so prolific a source of confusion in the study of any subject, that it seems wise to reduce the nomenclature of version to such simplicity as is compatible with clearness.

Cephalic version indicates that some other position has been changed so that the head presents.

Pelvic version indicates that some other position has been changed so that the breech presents. Podalic version is a term which should be included under the head of pelvic version, inasmuch as it is but a step farther in that procedure.

Internal rotation of the child is the term which signifies that, while the long axis of the child bears the same relationship to the long axis of the uterus, the occiput has been made to undergo a half-rotation.

This changing of the foetal relationship to the uterine may be accomplished in three ways: External, internal, or combined external and internal manipulation. Hence, to sum up this simplification of the nomenclature as applied to version, it may be taken for granted that all versions are either cephalic, pelvic, or internal rotation of the child, and that the operation is performed either by external, internal, or combined external and internal manipulation.

Cephalic version has found a few advocates and, theoretically, should be performed in all breech or transverse presentations where no complications exist to contra-indicate such a procedure. Pinard, who perhaps has done more than any other to popularize cephalic version, intimates that any other than a head presentation is due to some abnormal accommodation between the head and the pelvic inlet. Granting this to be true, it would seem that this very fact would contra-indicate the operation. So rarely will the patient be able to deliver herself, even after the cephalic version has been performed, that the operation is not to be regarded as practical except in a very limited number of cases.

Almost the only condition which renders cephalic version practicable is in transverse positions, where the waters have not escaped. The operation is contra-indicated in all cases where a rapid termination of the labor is indicated, when the child is not freely movable *in utero,* and in prolapse of the cord. Should the operation be determined upon in cases of transverse position, as indicated above, the combined method of Braxton Hicks is far more likely to be successful than either the external or internal alone. Chloroform anaesthesia should be produced and the patient placed on a table which has been properly covered and protected. The operator and his assistant must exercise absolute care in cleansing their hands and arms. The patient's bladder should be emptied and a rectal enema given. The external genitals and vagina should be cleansed with soap and water by means of a brush and afterward douched with some antiseptic solution, such as bichloride-of-mercury solution 1 to 1000, or creolin solution 1 to 100. The prone lithotomy position will, perhaps, render the operation least difficult. The patient being in the condition of surgical anaesthesia, the operator proceeds to carefully palpate the abdomen and determine the position of the child. The operator now redisinfects his hand and, selecting the one which he most frequently uses in making vaginal examinations, introduces the hand into the vagina. If the os is dilated sufficiently to admit the first and second fingers, they are carefully passed through the cervix, using as little force as is possible, so that the membranes may not be ruptured. If the os is not dilated it will be necessary to gradually introduce one finger, and, as soon as possible, the second. By slowly separating the fingers as much as possible enough room can soon be gained so that the fingers can be passed into the uterus. Should a contraction of the uterus take place the operator will desist from any manipulation in order that the integrity of the membranes may not be endangered. The fingers now seek the presenting part, and if it be a shoulder it is gradually raised and pushed toward the breech. The assistant at the same time pushes the head toward the pelvic inlet, while with the other hand the operator governs the movements of the breech, pushing it up toward the fundus. As soon as the head impinges on the vaginal fingers it may be made to settle into the brim of the pelvis. Carefully controlling the body of the child so that it may not again assume the transverse position, the membranes are ruptured and the water allowed to escape. This permits the uterus to contract more firmly on the body of the child, and thus retains the head in its proper position. The remainder of the delivery may now be left to nature unless some further indication presents itself.

Pelvic version is, as already stated, the term applied to the operation of converting some other into a breech presentation. It is of no advantage unless the operator goes a step farther and brings down a foot, thus performing a podalic version. This operation, considered from an elective stand-point, and not as a measure of last resort, is capable of producing more favorable results than has ever been credited to it. It is not fair to charge this operation with fatal results to mother or child when the operation has been resorted to only after repeated vain attempts to deliver the child with forceps, or after the mother has become exhausted with her long-continued efforts to overcome a resistance greater than the force at her disposal. In the hands of one who recognizes the difficulties to be overcome, either at the beginning of the labor or soon afterward, it becomes a powerful measure in saving lives. Podalic version is indicated (1) in transverse presentations where the child is not freely movable, or when cephalic version is not indicated; (2) in head presentations where, from some complication, the head fails to engage; (3) hi cases where it becomes necessary to expedite the delivery while the head is yet above the brim of the pelvis; (4) in head presentations where the safety of the mother or the child is likely to be endangered should the head be allowed to enter the pelvic canal.

The indication for podalic rather than cephalic version in transverse presentations will be found far more frequent, inasmuch as these cases are not always diagnosed in that stage of the labor which makes cephalic version possible. If the head is still above the brim of the pelvis and *movable,* podalic version is so much less dangerous than delivery by forceps that it should be adopted. Even in the hands of the most expert the application of high forceps is fraught with no small danger to the integrity of the soft parts of the mother.

In that class of cases where it becomes necessary to expedite the delivery, such as eclampsia, placenta previa, accidental haemorrhage, or pressure on the prolapsed cord, podalic version is the operation which yields the very best results.

The danger of allowing certain malpositions of head presentations to enter the pelvic canal as such is so well known and admitted that they need but little more than be mentioned. In face presentations and in occipito-posterior positions which cannot be corrected by internal rotation, podalic version should be performed.

Podalic version is contra-indicated (1) when the cervix is not dilated or dilatable; (2) when the uterus is in tetanic spasm around the foetus; (3) when the presenting part has become so firmly wedged into the pelvic inlet that undue force is necessary to push it upward; (4) in contracted pelves when the conjugate is less than three inches and three-quarters, and in oblique contractions when the brim of the pelvis is seriously encroached upon.

Operators who disregard the first contra-indication are the ones who will most frequently be compelled to perform craniotomy on the after-coming head which has been grasped in a partially-dilated cervix. This, of course, applies when extraction follows version immediately. The combined method permits version with but slight dilatation of the cervix.

When the uterus is in tetanic spasm around the foetus the operation is fraught with so much danger that it is not advisable. Long-continued dry labors or the injudicious use of ergot is the most frequent cause of this condition, and rupture of the uterus is too possible an occurrence.

If the presenting part has become firmly impacted the force necessary to dislodge it will endanger the integrity of the soft parts so much that the operation is inadvisable, and some less dangerous method must be adopted.

Although it is easy to turn the child in cases where the pelvis is contracted, yet the delivery of a living child is so uncertain if the conjugate is less than three inches and threequarters that it becomes a contra-indication to podalic version. Perhaps one of the most frequent causes of failure in saving the life of the child in podalic version is the neglect on the part of the operator to take careful pelvic measurements.

It is not meant that the physician must leave his patient and seek a pelvimeter of some peculiar pattern, but it is meant that with his ringers he can form so nearly an exact idea of the true conjugate that he will be able to depend upon it. (The details for doing this have already been given under the head of pelvimetry.)

In this, as in all other obstetric operations, it is absolutely necessary that an exact diagnosis should be made.

The operator must have a true mental picture of the position of the foetus *in utero.* As stated under the head of cephalic version, external palpation and vaginal examination will, in most cases, render the diagnosis clear; but it is not infrequent, even in the most skilled hands, to make a mistake if these two methods alone are resorted to. If there is any doubt it is better to put the patient thoroughly under the influence of chloroform and introduce the *hand* into the vagina and two fingers into the uterus. In head presentations the ear becomes a most valuable landmark. If it is felt, it is with perfect ease that even one of no great experience can determine the position of the head. Let it be remembered that in but very few cases is there necessity for haste in making a careful examination. It is only after extraction begins that work must be rapid.

Before operating, the physician must have a *personal* knowledge that all the necessary preparations for the various emergencies which may arise are at hand.

Fluid extract of ergot and the usual restoratives,—whisky, strychnia tablets, etc.,—together with an hypodermatic syringe in good working-order, should be in readiness. A perfectly clean, preferably new, gravity syringe, with an intra-uterine glass nozzle, should be filled with some mild antiseptic solution which is heated to 118 F. (Creolin solution 1 to 100 and bichloride-of-mercury solution 1 to 10,000 are as good as any.) Basins of hot and cold water and a number of freshly-laundried towels should be in the room. Iodoform gauze 10 per cent., which is known to be fresh and clean, for intra-uterine tamponade, should be cut in strips several yards long and two inches wide. A basin of some antiseptic solution and a new nail-brush should be in easy reach of the operator-. A shorthandled forceps, in case the after-coming head becomes arrested at the brim, should be sterilized. Needles, needle-holder, silk, silk-worm-gut ligatures, sponge-holders, and artery-clamps should be boiled and placed in a tray of sterilized water. The operator and his assistants must be conscientious in the details of antisepsis. If no operating-gown is at hand, a folded sheet can be made to take its place. The hands and nails are rendered clean with soap and brush and afterward by *immersion* in bichloride-of-mercury solution 1 to 1000 for at least five minutes.

The patient should be thoroughly anaesthetized and transferred from the bed to any ordinary table, which has been covered with a blanket and a piece of rubber sheeting. The patient should be placed on her back and the buttocks drawn well over the edge of the table. The knees are to be separated and drawn up over the abdomen. Confining the knees in this position by means of an improvised crutch made by tying one end of a sheet around one of the knees, passing the sheet back of the patient's head and tying the remaining knee with the other end of the sheet will leave more hands free and necessitate a less number of assistants.

The vulva and adjacent parts should be thoroughly cleansed with soap, water, and brush, and afterward with some antiseptic solution.

The catheter should be introduced, even though the patient may have recently passed her water. It is wise for the operator to inform his assistants exactly what duty is to be performed by each. It is possible to perform this operation simply with the help of one physician and a nurse, or some one who will act in that capacity; but it is far better to have the assistance of two physicians,—one whose sole duty it will be to administer the anaesthetic, and the other to assist directly in the operation. In regard to the hand which the operator should use in performing podalic version, it should be borne in mind that if an extremity is to be grasped the palmar surface of the hand must be turned toward the abdomen of the child. If the back of the child is to the left, the left hand is to be used; if to the right, the right hand must be used. From the variableness of the position of the child, the physician should attempt to educate both hands to an equal degree of tactile sensibility.

As has been stated previously, version may be performed by three methods,—external, internal, and the combined external and internal.

Pelvic version by the external method is so seldom applicable that little need be said of it. It is not often applicable, from the fact that a substitution of a breech for a head presentation is scarcely ever a desired condition. It is not often practical, inasmuch as the great majority of the indications for version presupposes the determination for rapid delivery by bringing down a foot. In transverse presentations when the waters have not ruptured, and when the breech is nearer the pelvic brim than the head, it may be indicated. While it may be in its performance absolutely without danger to the mother, it must be remembered that it may put the cord to such a disadvantage that the child's life will be jeopardized.

If this method is decided upon, the patient should be placed upon her back with her knees drawn up so that the abdominal walls may be relaxed. The operator stands to the side of and facing the patient. The exact position of the child should be mapped out. The physician then places one hand over the buttocks and the other over the head of the child, and, by pulling the buttocks toward him and pushing the head up, he attempts to convert the position first into a transverse and then into a breech presentation. If the presentation is already a transverse, and the breech is nearer the brim, the head may be raised as the breech is forced into the pelvis. It is necessary that manipulations be made only during the interim between pains, and during the contractions of the uterus an attempt should be made only to retain the amount of advantage gained. This method presupposes relaxed abdominal walls, unruptured membranes, and free mobility of the child.

The combined method made so famous by the name of Braxton Hicks, who perfected and popularized it, is likewise limited in its application, inasmuch as it is not often successful, unless the liquor amnii is still present or has only recently escaped, and where considerable mobility of the child is still present. It is seldom performed, since version is nearly always followed by immediate extraction, and this presupposes sufficient dilatation to admit of the entire hand being introduced into the uterus.

In certain cases of placenta praevia where haemorrhage is taking place before the cervix is very much dilated, the combined method is of great advantage. In such cases the prime object is to control the haemorrhage, and if the operator can succeed in introducing even two fingers into the uterus he may be able to draw down a foot and thus plug the cervix with the buttocks. The operation is not easy or advisable if the head is wedged in the pelvis, nor when the uterus is contracted around the child. The patient should be thoroughly under the influence of the anaesthetic and the buttocks drawn over the edge of the table, as has been described.

After thorough asepsis on the part of the operator and his assistants and the external genitals and vagina of the patient, the entire hand, which has previously been dipped into 1 to 100 creolin solution, and corresponding to the position of the occiput, folded upon itself cone-shape, should be introduced into the vagina. All force imparted to the hand should be gentle and at first directed downward and backward, then forward and upward, till the cervix is felt.

Counter-pressure with the unemployed hand can be made over the fundus of the uterus by the operator better than any skilled assistant can do for him. This counter-pressure answers two purposes: the vaginal attachment to the uterus is not put on an undue amount of strain and the cervix is forced nearer the examining finger.

If one finger only can be introduced, proceed to dilate with the index finger, if previous dilatation has not taken place (Fig.

As soon as two fingers can be introduced the head is sought and pushed up toward the side to which the occiput is directed, while with the other hand the buttocks are brought down in the opposite direction. If extension of the head has taken place the chest of the child will be felt, which should be pushed upward in the same way as in case the head is felt. As soon as the head is raised beyond the reach of the fingers the knees are sought, which should now be within reach. The knee must be carefully distinguished from the elbow before traction is made upon it. There will be no difficulty in doing this if the operator remembers that the flexed elbow points toward the buttocks and the flexed knee points toward the head. It is not necessary to waste time looking for the patella; it is difficult to recognize, and the above rule is accurate. If the knee is felt, it should be grasped (Fig. 46) between the two fingers and brought still lower toward the brim; at the same time the other hand can now be used to push the head toward the fundus. As the knee is brought down the fingers can be made to slip down the leg until the foot is grasped and extracted (Fig. 47).

It sometimes happens that the foot is felt before the knee; if so, the position of the great toe and the malleoli will enable the physician to distinguish the foot from the hand. If the foot is felt and recognized it should be brought down, thus completing the version.

It has already been said that the external method and the combined method of Braxton Hicks are limited in their applications for the reasons stated.

It is the internal method which has the broadest field of application, and which is of incalculable value in certain cases.

The indications and contra-indications have already been given. The position of the patient and the previous preparations are the same as in the external method. This operation should not be performed until the cervix is fully dilated or dilatable. Under thorough aseptic precautions the hand is introduced into the vagina very gently, until the cervix is reached. If the cervix is not dilated, its dilatation should be at once begun. By introducing one finger into the cervix it is easy to determine whether any constricting ring exists around the os. If such is found to be the case, and it does not soon yield to the finger, it is wise, in case of urgency, to expedite the dilatation by using the knife. Any blunt-pointed bistoury, which has been protected by wrapping a piece of gauze around the blade so that only one-half inch at the point is left free, may be used.

Using the fingers as a guide, the knife protected in this way may be passed into the os and six or eight slight nicks made into the hardened ring of the cervix, distributed throughout its circumference. It is not necessary that the cuts be more than an eighth of an inch in depth. It will astonish one who has not tried this little procedure how much this will facilitate the dilatation. Under gentle pressure two, and sometimes three, fingers can be introduced and the dilatation completed. If the liquor amnii has not previously escaped, care should be exercised during the dilatation that the fingers do not make undue pressure on the membranes; for it is better, if possible, to have the membranes intact until the cervix is fully dilated. This procedure of manually dilating the cervix, while simple, is oftentimes most trying on the operator's powers of endurance, and frequently he will be forced to delegate a part of its performance to his assistant. The hand should be redisinfected with creolin solution 1 to 100, which at the same time takes the place of other lubricants, whenever there is occasion to introduce it into the vagina.

When the os is fully dilated the operator should pass that hand which corresponds to the position of the occiput (right hand if the occiput is turned to the right) into the uterus, and if the membranes aie still intact rupture them. The movements of the hand must be gentle and *between* pains. If a contraction of the uterus should take place, the hand must be flattened out and held perfectly still until it has subsided. The head is pushed to one side and a foot is sought, and as soon as it is recognized it should be grasped (Fig. 48). Before traction is made on the foot it is wise to note whether the cord is looped over the leg; if so, it must be released. While the cord is between the fingers its pulsations should be noted as regards their frequency and character, for this may give the operator additional reason for hastening the delivery.

. As the foot is drawn down the other hand is placed over the fundus and makes counter-pressure. It should be the duty of the assistant to govern the movements of the head, and as

Fig. 49.—Completing the Version.

soon as the operator makes traction on the foot he should attempt to carry the head in the opposite direction.

As the operator draws the foot down into the vagina, the head ascends to the fundus and the version is completed (Fig. 49).

In transverse presentations, if there is no prolapse of the arm, the same method is to be adopted for performing version as has been described above, except, as the head is already above the brim, a foot is sought at once.

In cases where the arm has prolapsed, but has not become impacted, it can be pushed up with but little difficulty. It is well, however, while the arm is still in reach, to fasten a loop of tape around the wrist before it is pushed up. This will be of assistance during the extraction, for, by drawing gently on the tape, at least that arm will be prevented from becoming extended.

In those cases where the arm has become prolapsed and long-continued uterine contractions have taken place, the thorax may have become wedged into the pelvic outlet. It must be

Fig. 50.—Impacted Shoulder.

borne in mind that here it will be necessary to replace that part which last came down before the arm and shoulder can be replaced (Fig. 50). The thorax must be carried up above the brim before any attempt is made to replace the arm. This procedure requires the greatest care on the part of the physician, or else a ruptured uterus is almost certain to result. If, after making well-directed pressure from below with firm counterpressure over the fundus, the impaction cannot be relieved, it is better to discontinue the efforts to perform version, and either do embryotomy in the interest of the mother or, if the mother be in good condition and the outlook for saving the child not too poor, resort to symphysiotomy.

The indications for version almost always presuppose immediate delivery.

Much has been written on the subject, " Which foot should be drawn down?" If there is no immediate reason for haste and the operator has time to make his selection, it would seem that it is best to draw down that foot which is nearest the anterior surface of uterus. In actual work, however, it does not make much difference which foot is brought down. That

Fig. 51.—Introduction of the Left Hand to Bring down the Posterior (Left) Leg.

one is usually best which can be soonest recognized and most firmly grasped (Plate VI).

It is better, in primiparae certainly, and often in multiparee, that one foot only be brought down, for the cervix which has permitted a half-breech to escape will be less likely to grasp the after-coming head than if it has been dilated by the pelvis alone. If, however, traction on one leg does not prove successful, it will be necessary to draw down the other (Fig. 51 and Plate VII). As the foot emerges from the vulva it is to be wrapped in a warm towel, which not only offers a better grasp on the part, but also tends to prevent the cool air of the room from causing enough reflex irritation to establish respiratory efforts on the part of the child. Soon the leg can be grasped in the same way, and at this time traction is to be made in the axis of the brim downward (Fig. 52).

It is very necessary that during the entire process of extraction the assistant, should make well-directed pressure on the child's head. This tends to prevent extension of the head and also furnishes the *vis a tergo* which the patient, by reason of the deep anaesthesia, cannot give.

As the buttocks emerge from the vulva, one finger of the hand corresponding to the flexed thigh should be hooked into the groin; this will enable the operator to lessen the traction on the extended leg, and at the same time permit him to exert greater tractile force. By raising the buttocks and making traction upward the flexed thigh can be made to clear the vulva. The pelvis should now be grasped with both hands and drawn downward again in the axis of the brim.

As the cord comes down it is to be drawn upon from the *placental* side, and if it is over one of the legs it must be released (Fig. 53) and placed in the most favorable position as regards pressure. In rare instances it will be impossible to draw the cord down without making undue traction. If such should prove to be the case, it should be secured by means of two artery-clamps and cut. Of course, if tins is done, it will be necessary to hasten the delivery as much as possible.

When the scapulae appear the arms must be liberated before extraction is continued. Under favorable circumstances, —that is, if the assistant has kept up intelligent pressure on the fundus, or if the cervix was fully dilated previous to the version, or if the operator has not made traction in too rapid a manner,—the arms will be folded on the chest and their extraction will be easy.

Even in the hands of the best operators and with the best assistants the arms sometimes become unavoidably extended. Although their extraction must be accomplished in as rapid a manner as possible, there is no need of breaking the arm if care is taken.

The arm which is to the rear is usually more easily liberated. To do this the operator seizes the legs with one hand and carries the child's body well upward. This will cause the posterior shoulder to be more readily reached, and will permit more room for the manipulations necessary. Two fingers of the disengaged hand are passed over the back and posterior shoulder (Fig. 54). The shoulder can now be pulled down gently so that the arm may be more easily felt. As soon as the humerus is felt it is to be pushed forward and toward the opposite shoulder. Now, by drawing the humerus downward the arm becomes flexed at the elbow and the forearm rests on the chest of the child. Its extraction after this is simple, and the same as in unextended cases. If it is impossible to extract the arm in this way, the operator should pass the palmar surface of his hand over the abdomen of the child and attempt to hook one finger over the elbow of the posterior arm, and by gentle traction flex it over the chest (Plate VIII).

After the posterior arm has been liberated, the child's body should be carried downward, and the anterior arm is rarely difficult of extraction. Should, however, there be any trouble in releasing it, the anterior shoulder is to be rotated to the rear, where, with more room, its extraction is simple.

With the arms released the operator hastens to extract the head.

If firm pressure has been maintained on the fundus the head should be found in the pelvis, either straight or somewhat flexed.

Extraction of the head may be accomplished either manually or instrumental!'. Inasmuch as less danger to both child and mother results from manual extraction, forceps on the after-coming head should be left as a last resort.

If there is no great disproportion between the head and the pelvic outlet, extraction will not be difficult.

The child's body should be wrapped in a warm towel. Grasping the pelvis, with his left hand placed underneath the child and allowing the legs to straddle over his arm, the operator seizes the child's neck with his right hand, the palmar surface of the hand being over the shoulders of the child and the neck between the middle and third fingers (Fig. 55). Firm traction is now made almost directly downward. When the occiput has engaged immediately behind the pubic arch, the child's body is to be carried directly upward (Fig. 56). In favorable cases, the face, brow, and head will sweep over the perineum and extraction will be complete. So easy an extraction as this is the exception, however, from the very fact that those cases which demand version usually presuppose a disproportion between the size of the head and of the pelvic canal. When such is the case, other manipulations are necessary. The operator, as in the preceding method, lets the child's body rest on his left arm. The middle and index fingers of the left hand are passed into the vagina until the fingers can be applied on either side of the child's nose, the tips of the fingers resting over the malar prominences. Traction is made with this hand downward, while with the right hand the occiput is pushed upward and forward. This manipulation has the tendency to flex the head. As soon as flexion is accomplished, the operator grasps the child's neck with his right hand in the manner described above, and now

Fig. 56.—The Child is Lifted Over the Perineum ami the Occiput Passes from

Under the Symphysis.

with both hands makes firm and continued traction. The left hand should remain over the malar prominences, and not be introduced into the child's mouth, if firm traction is to be made with that hand. Traction with the finger in the mouth does not produce flexion to the same degree, and if much force is used fracture of the jaw will probably be produced. If, however, the delivery is very difficult and prolonged, if any convulsive movements of the child indicate an attempt at respiration, or if the pulsations of the cord are becoming imperceptible, a most valuable procedure is to introduce two fingers into the child's mouth, and by slightly separating them permit air to enter the child's mouth, so that respiration may be established. The right hand must now be depended upon to make the necessary traction to complete the delivery (Plate IX).

If the head become arrested at the brim, extraction is far more difficult. Here the feet must be grasped with the left hand and the right fingers placed so as to straddle the nape of the neck, and traction is to be made directly downward. At the same time the assistant makes firm pressure from above, forcing the head downward (Plate X). Should the head fail to descend, it will often do so if it is made to enter the brim in a transverse position. To do this, the operator, in place of making traction while the back of child is directed upward, turns the entire body of the child so that the back is directed to the side which corresponds with the shoulder that was posterior. (If the left shoulder was posterior, the back of the child should be turned toward the left side of the pelvis.) Now, by making traction directly downward, the head will enter the brim through its greatest diameter and descend into the lesser pelvis. Traction now will usually result in the occiput turning forward, when extraction may be completed as described before.

Should the occiput not rotate forward, then the perineum, instead of the symphysis, becomes the fulcrum, and downward traction will cause the face and brow to sweep under the symphysis and delivery is completed (Plate XI).

In case, however, extension has taken place and the chin becomes arrested behind the symphysis (Fig. 57), traction should be made upward and two fingers of one hand should be passed into the rectum and the occiput " shelled" out over the perineum.

When all these means have been tried and failed, forceps should be applied. The authors have obtained better results with the short-handle Hunter forceps than any other used. Usually the forceps can be adjusted posteriorly (Fig. 58 and Plate XII) better and more quickly than anteriorly, but it should be applied to that aspect of the child which can be most rapidly reached. It should be applied to the sides of the pelvis regardless of the position of the child's head.

It must be remembered that after extraction of the arms the head must be delivered within three to five minutes if a living child is to be obtained. It is true that in exceptional cases a living child may be extracted within fifteen minutes, but this is very rare. Care must be exercised that the forceps does not slip during extraction, or else grave injury will result to both mother and child.

As has been stated before, internal rotation of the foetus is an operation which must be included in the consideration of versions, for the operation consists in turning the child in its long axis. This operation is indicated only in occipito-posterior positions, while the head is yet movable above the brim. The operation should not be performed if the head has firmly engaged, nor if the waters have drained away, nor if for any reason the labor must be hastily terminated. If the waters have already drained away and the uterus is firmly contracted around the child, it will be necessary to apply forceps and hope for rotation in the descent. In the great majority of cases this rotation will ensue. If there is any reason to hastily terminate the labor, it is better to perform podalic version and extract. An occipito-posterior position is, as a rule, associated with slow engagement, and this is often the first factor which attracts the attention of the obstetrician to the fact that the labor is not a normal one. The physician often makes his first examination in a somewhat perfunctory way,—that is, he satisfies himself that the head is presenting, and perhaps determines that the cervix is slowly dilating. If such has been his course, and if after several hours repeated examination shows but little increase in the dilatation of the cervix, or that the head does not engage even under the influence of firm uterine contractions, he should at once determine what conditions are present which are prolonging the first stage.

An examination with one or two fingers introduced into the vagina, even conjoined with abdominal palpation, will often not result in the information necessary to determine this point. Certainly it will not if the patient is nervous and resists the physician's efforts. An anaesthetic should be administered if satisfactory results are to be obtained from the examination.

The preparation of the patient and the operator should be the same as for podalic version. The operator introduces that hand into the vagina which he is in the habit of using when making a vaginal examination. If the cervix is dilated so that two fingers can be passed into the uterus, no further dilatation will be necessary at this time. The head should be carefully raised between pains, and no undue pressure made upon the membranes. The fontanelles are sought and examined. If any doubt of the real position remain after this, the ear should be felt; this will be an unfailing guide.

If the occiput is posterior the cervix should be dilated, preparatory to performing the internal rotation, in the same way as has been described for podalic version. With the cervix fully dilated the hand is introduced into the uterus. If the head has slightly engaged, it should be gently pushed up. The fœtus is now grasped and slowly rotated in its long axis until the occiput is anterior. The hand should now be slowly withdrawn until the head can be grasped, and in this position the operator waits for uterine contraction. When this has occurred the head is driven down and engagement ensues. It is wise to retain the hand until two or three contractions have taken place, so that the head may be firmly engaged. The case may now be left to nature, or, if necessity demands, the forceps may be applied and extraction completed (Plate XIII).

The course of action herein advocated is not novel, nor is it as radical as at first sight it may appear. The management of occipito-posterior positions has for a long time been a matter of strife among obstetricians. The lever, the forceps applied inversely, podalic version, the conversion into a face presentation,—such means from time to time have been advocated. When the occiput, in faulty position, has become impacted, certain of these measures are forced upon us, with consequent damage to the woman and with as yet not sufficiently recognized injury to the fœtal brain.

For the purpose of rotation nothing can take the place of the *aseptic* hand, aside from the fact that at one and the same

Method of Grasping the Child-s Body in Performing Internal Rotation. time the hand may detect any additional anomaly hitherto unsuspected, such as pelvic deformity, which, aside from being a further cause of slow or impossible engagement, may alter the field of election at the very best time (from the stand-point of both the woman and the fœtus),—that is to say, when the conditions are still favorable for version or some other procedure.

When the occiput rotates backward into the hollow of the sacrum, we are face to face with what—there is uniform agreement—constitutes one of the most difficult cases in obstetrics. The clean, educated obstetric hand at the pelvic brim is a source of positive safety to both the mother and child, compared with waiting until exhaustion calls for, for instance, the forceps within the pelvic brim.

A tedious first stage, characterized by short, nagging pains, is a fairly-uniform accompaniment of the instances which should cause anxiety. It seems clear that *manual* examination at this time will often lead to the adoption of a procedure which will alter the prognosis of, and lessen the difficulties attendant upon, the persistent oblique and sacro-rotated occipital position.

Prognosis.—Naturally the prognosis will vary greatly according to the conditions demanding the operation. In those cases where retraction of the uterus has not taken place, and where there exists no disproportion between the head and pelvis, the prognosis for the mother should be absolutely good if the operation is performed under aseptic precautions and in a skillful manner. The same may be said of the child if the operation is undertaken before the fœtal heart shows signs of failure. In the proportion, however, that these favorable conditions decrease will the mortality rate to the child increase. There should be no mortality at any time for the mother unless uterine retraction has taken place, the operation being done only as a last resort, or where the pelvic outlet is markedly disproportionate to the fœtal head. CHAPTER V. SYMPHYSIOTOMY.

The operation of symphysiotomy was first performed in the year 1777 by Jean Rene Sigault. After a protracted convalescence the ultimate result was successful, and this led other operators to test the procedure. The results, however, were not sufficiently favorable to lead to its general adoption, as shown by the fact that up to the year 1858 the operation was performed only 86 times, with the loss of 29 women and the extraction alive of 29 children. The operation thence fell into disuse until the year 1866, when it was revived in Naples by Morrisani and Novi. Outside of Italy, however, the operation attracted scarcely any attention, receiving but scant, if any, reference in works on obstetrics until the year 1890, when, largely through the publications of Pinard, of Paris, and Harris, of Philadelphia, the attention of obstetricians was attracted to the really beneficent results which were being secured through timely resort to it. The unfavorable results from the operation during its early years were unquestionably due to the lack of appreciation of the necessity of both asepsis and of election, and therefore our study of the operation need be based purely on the results which are yielded in modern times, when both of these factors play the chief role in obstetric surgery.

In 1892 Harris collated the operations which had been performed from January, 1886, up to July, 1892, as follows: 44 operations, with one maternal death and the loss of 4 children. Up to this time the operation had never been performed in the United States, although practical obstetricians had been giving much attention to another alternate operation having in view the avoidance of embryotomy,—the Caesarean section. From this date on, however, as if by magic, operations were reported from various sections of the country until we are now in the position of being able to judge the operation from the stand-point of home results. Meanwhile, Pinard, in Paris, has been equally active, and the number of recorded operations has reached a sufficiently large basis to admit even of a degree of dogmatism in the estimation of the proper sphere of symphysiotomy. The inevitable result of the rapid acceptance of the operation has been, as will be noted, a higher mortality rate,— in a measure doubtless due to the inexpertness of the majority of operators performing their first of the kind.

Indications and Limitations.—The aim of the operation of symphysiotomy is, through section of the pubic joint, to allow of separation of the symphysis, whereby the pelvic diameters are widened sufficiently to enable the delivery, *per vias naturales,* of a fœtus which otherwise would have to be sacrificed. The operation, then, is performed purely in the interests of the child, taking the place of embryotomy and displacing the Caesarean section from the stand-point of the relative indications. Before the resuscitation of symphysiotomy, indeed, the alternative was either mutilation of the fœtus or the subjection of the woman to the major operation of abdominal section..When, therefore, symphysiotomy becomes, as it should, an elective operation, with consequent lowering of the maternal mortality rate to *nil,* there will exist, other things equal, no further call for embryotomy, and the Caesarean section will be reserved strictly for cases which fall under the absolute indication. It is significant, indeed, that more than one obstetrician in Europe is already on record as claiming that the time has definitely arrived when the physician is not called upon to sacrifice the living fœtus. In the United States, however, the time is not ripe for such an extreme statement outside of maternity hospitals. In private practice the woman herself or her representative must continue to exercise the right of choice until the mortality rate from symphysiotomy has fallen to a figure at least as low as in expert hands is associated with embryotomy.

Through experiment on the cadaver we have learned that when the pubic symphysis is cut and the knees of the cadaver are separated the pubic bones diverge, without inflicting damage on the sacro-iliac joints, to the extent of two and three-fourths to three inches. Into the opening formed in front the presenting part of the foetus may enter and the following space is gained in the various diameters of the pelvis. The true conjugate increases to the extent of from one-fourth to one-half an inch and the transverse and oblique diameters gain from threefourths to one and a half inches. It is at once apparent how, with a fcetus of average size, this operation enables delivery to be accomplished without mutilation of the foetus, since the gain in the pelvic dimensions applies with equal force to the types of deformed pelves most frequently met with,—the flat and the generally contracted.

The indications for the operation are as follow: The consent of the woman or her representative. The foetus viable and the woman and the foetus not exhausted through protracted labor. Careful precedent pelvimetry, instrumental and manual, proving that there exists dystocia which will not yield to either version or the forceps and testifying to the existence of a type of pelvis where, after pubic section, the sacro-iliac synchondroses will yield. In the generally contracted pelvis the conjugata vera must be at least three and three-fourths inches in dimensions, and in the flat pelvis, where it will be borne in mind the transverse diameter is relatively wide, the conjugata vera may be reduced even to two and three-fourths inches if the child is below the average size. In impacted occipito-posterior positions and in irreducible face presentations. The cervix must be dilated or dilatable. The presence of ankylosis of one or the other sacro-iliac joint must be ruled out.

Before passing to a consideration of the technique of the operation, it is well to recall, briefly the structures involved in the operation and to point out the risks to which the maternal structures are subjected. In the vast majority of women at or near term there exists normally a certain amount of separation at the symphysis, provided this be not ankylosed, when, of course, the operation is *per se* contra-indicated. The operation is entirely extra-peritoneal, the bladder stripped of the peritoneum, and the urethra lying immediately under the symphysis. In certain instances, however, as Dickinson, of Brooklyn, reminds us, the peritoneum pouches downward, and there may be danger of injuring this.

As a rule, however, the bladder and the urethra are the only organs which are likely to be injured, and these, we will show, need not be if the requisite care is taken during the performance of the operation and afterward when the parts are brought together. We are speaking now, of course, of the

Fig. 59.—The Bulging of Peritoneum and of Bladder into the
Opening at the Joint.
subcutaneous performance of the operation, the method which is favored by most practical accoucheurs. The open method of operating involves the structures and the vessels which cover the anterior face of the pubes, and the selection of this method of operating converts symphysiotomy into a much more serious operation and complicates greatly convalescence as well.

The two factors which control the result of this operation are *election* and *aaepticism*. Where the operation is indicated it should be performed in a timely manner, and to-day there is no excuse for inattention to the stringent rules of cleanliness whereby the surgery of the present is so sharply differentiated from that of the past. If but one lesson has been taught by the results secured during the past three years, it is that symphysiotomy need not have a mortality rate. As will be noted later, the fatal cases resulting since the rejuvenation of the operation have been due either to the fact that the operation has been performed on an exhausted woman, or else because, through inattention to asepsis, the woman has succumbed to septicaemia.

The instruments essential for the performance of the operation are: a stout, blunt-pointed bistoury, a few artery-forceps, a needle-holder, needles, a metallic catheter, or a metal sound. Silkworm gut forms the preferable material for sutures. The Galbiati knife, which is highly favored by the Italians, has been found unnecessary. Indeed, in certain cases, the use of this instrument is dangerous to the integrity of the maternal parts, if resort to it be at all possible.

In certain exceptional instances the symphysis of the pubes deviates from the mid-line, and in others the union of the halves is not cartilaginous, but bony. When this untoward complication is present it will be impossible to separate the symphysis with a knife, and a chain-saw is requisite. Fortunately, this occurrence is a rarity; still, the physician should be prepared for every emergency, and, therefore, should add a saw to his armamentarium. t *Technique of the Operation.*—The method of operating which is favored by the vast majority of those who have had practical experience is the subcutaneous one. There are weighty reasons why the open method should be rejected. If this is selected it will be very difficult to avoid infecting the wound with lochia during convalescence, and, further, the tissues near the clitoris are peculiarly vascular,—all the more so during pregnancy,—and section made in this neighborhood exposes the woman to the risk of c onsiderable haemorrhage of a type very difficult to control. There are a sufficient number of modern instances of the operation on record now, where the subcutaneous method was followed, to prove its perfect feasibility, and in certain cases its wonderful simplicity. Although trained assistants are helpful, their presence is not strictly requisite.

The woman having been anaesthetized, the abdomen is prepared as for an abdominal section,—that is to say, the pubes are carefully shaved and thoroughly disinfected. The bladder is emptied. An incision is made in the mid-line down to the recti muscles, beginning at the suprapubic eminence, and extending upward lor about three inches. The recti are separated by the ringer and the handle of the scalpel, and this brings us to the retropubic space. A catheter is now inserted into the bladder and handed to an assistant to depress the urethra from under the pubes. This is a highly important step, since one of the accidents associated with the performance of symphysiotomy is injury to the neck of the bladder. The accident is entirely avoidable, and much depends, therefore, on the assistant who holds this catheter. The operator's index finger is next inserted under the symphysis to further protect the bladder, and it must be held there until the section of the pubic symphysis is completed. If the foetal presenting part has not as yet engaged, or, in case it has, if the part can be pressed upward, the inserting of the finger is easy, and there remains further space for the Galbiati knife if the operator prefer it; but in case of engagement of the foetal part it will be found difficult to insert the finger, and, this accomplished, there is scant room, if any, for the sickle-shaped knife. Hence the reason why later operators have discarded this knife and substituted the stout, bluntpointed bistoury. The linger being in place below the symphysis, the union of the pubic bones is incised in the direction from above downward and from without inward. The operator must not be satisfied until he has severed the inferior ligament of the pubes. If he fail to accomplish this the pubic bones simply separate at the top, and there is scant gain, if any, in the pelvic diametei-s. As soon as the subpubic ligament has been severed, the pubic bones separate and the pelvis becomes enlarged. As already noted, a separation of from two and onehalf to three inches is possible without inflicting damage on the sacro-iliac synchondroses. In order to avoid separation beyond this, an assistant on either side of the woman should make firm inward pressure on the trochanters whilst delivery is being effected.

Any haemorrhage occurring during the steps of the operation should, if arterial, be checked by torsion or ligature. Venous oozing, which is apt to be considerable, is met by the tampon with sterilized gauze. This tampon is left in place until delivery has been effected.

It has been claimed that after division of the symphysis delivery should be left to nature, except in instances where the condition of the woman or the foetus requires hasty action. There is, however, no advantage in this. The cervix being dilated or dilatable, since the woman is under anaesthesia, there is nothing to be gained by delay. If the head is above the brim, the membranes unruptured, or if the presenting part has just engaged and the membranes are intact, the conditions favorable for version are present and there is no valid reason why the physician should not proceed to deliver after this fashion. The chances are that the operation of symphysiotomy has been called for on account of maternal or of foetal dystocia, and under such condition, where version is possible, it should always be elected over the forceps. Where the presenting part has engaged, but cannot be delivered short of symphysiotomy, owing to contraction at the outlet, the forceps should be applied *lege artis*. If the operation of symphysiotomy has been elected to enable the delivery alive of a foetus presenting in a mentoposterior or in an occipito-posterior impacted position, then, after symphysiotomy, the malposition should be corrected as far as is feasible, and delivery be effected by the forceps.

After completion of the third stage of labor, the operator should turn his attention at once to the repair of the wound made necessary by the symphysiotomy. The aseptic catheter is again introduced into the bladder and handed to an assistant in order that the urethra and the bladder may be pressed downward carefully whilst the pubic bones are being brought into apposition. This step is a most important one. If neglected, or if carelessly performed, the bladder or urethra will be nipped in the symphysis, and in the course of a few days a fistula will be established. The thighs of the woman are rotated inward, and firm pressure is made on the trochanters by two assistants. The pubic bones are thus brought together, and are held there until the wound in the abdomen has been properly sutured and the bandage has been applied. If the subcutaneous operation has been performed, as we believe it should, it is useless to attempt to suture the symphysis. Nor is this necessary. Where the operation has been performed aseptically, and a proper bandage is applied, the pubic bones will remain in apposition and unite firmly. Unless the woman is specially fat, deep silk-worm-gut sutures will suffice for bringing together the abdominal wall. If the woman is stout it is preferable to unite the divided recti muscle by a running catgut suture and to treat the skin and fat by the open method, which insures, in such cases, firmer union. After the sutures are in position and the usual dressing has been applied, a wide strip of adhesive plaster, extending from the trochanters nearly to the umbilicus, is carried around the woman, whilst the assistants are maintaining firm pressure on the trochanters. Tins immobilizes the pelvis efficiently, and, barring indication of suppuration in the wound, this dressing need not be changed for from five to ten days. The after-treatment of the case is exactly similar to that which holds for the normal puerperium, except that very likely it will be necessary to catheterize the woman. The woman should be kept on her back for the first week, but after this period she may lie on her side. She should be kept in bed for at least three weeks, although cases have been allowed to rise sooner with apparently no bad effect. As a rule, in every woman, after symphysiotomy there will exist, for a variable interval, a greater or less degree of motion at the joint, but we question if this is greater than that which normally exists in young primiparffi after a difficult non-instrumental labor. The fact seems to have been overlooked that in probably the majority of gravid women there exists motion at the symphysis for a variable interval. This motion, however, is not associated with disability, and before very long the fibrous tissue becomes organized and motion cannot be detected. Even if there should remain a degree of separation at the symphysis after symphysiotomy, we should not look upon this as an evil, for in the event of a future pregnancy a second operation might not be demanded should the woman be allowed to go to term.

Complications.—In the reported modern cases, the only ones which need concern us, the most unfortunate complication noted has been the formation of a fistula of the urinary tract, either vaginal or abdominal. The essential step for avoiding this we have already laid stress upon. If, notwithstanding, the accident should occur, often the lesion will heal spontaneously under cleanliness and catheterization. If spontaneous repair should not occur, then, some time after the puerperium, a secondary operation will be called for. It is a noteworthy fact that fistulae have chiefly occurred in instances where the operation has been resorted to only after the foetal presenting part had become wedged in the pelvic brim, and where the Galbiati knife had been used. Ave believe that when it becomes the practice to elect the operation before engagement, or, at any rate, before futile attempts at engagement have necessarily resulted in more or less pressure on the neck of the bladder, this complication will become excessively infrequent. Further, we question if the use of the Galbiati knife, in cases where the presenting part has engaged, is not responsible for many of the fistulas. As we have already stated, when the presenting part has engaged there is scant room for the insertion of both the finger and the knife under the symphysis. The insertion of the finger is absolutely necessary in order to insure the safety of the bladder; the Galbiati knife is not necessary for the performance of the operation. The majority of operations in this country have been performed without this knife, and we would, therefore, limit its utility to instances where the foetal presenting part has not engaged, and where, therefore, there is ample room both for the ringer and the knife.

Haemorrhage as a complication of the operation need not be feared where the subcutaneous method is selected. At best this is only venous oozing, which is easily controlled by the gauze tampon. The open method of operating, which we do not indorse, entails, of course, wounding of the venous plexuses of the vestibule, as also the vessels which nourish the clitoris. Haemorrhage from this source may be very difficult to control, and the essential manipulations required carry extra chance of septicizing the woman. The open method of operating, then, should be strictly reserved for instances where deviation of the symphysis from the mid-line, or where the bony ankylosis forbids the performance of the operation by means of the knife, and calls for the chain-saw.

The further complication which is responsible for the loss of a fair percentage is septic infection,—a complication common to every surgical procedure, and an avoidable one.

When the operation was resuscitated it was feared that the ultimate result as regards locomotion would be bad. The record of the modern cases certifies, however, that this fear is unfounded. In many of the women there exists for a variable period a certain amount of motion at the joint, and in some cases the women complain of a sensation of motion there; but before long the fibrous tissue becomes organized, and these physical and rational symptoms disappear.

Prognosis.—For the purpose of determining statistically the prognosis of this operation, we shall consider alone the data which have accrued during the past few years. Prior to this period careless asepsis was responsible for a very high mortality rate.

The following data will enable us to judge the prognosis fairly: In general the mortality rate has varied from 8 to 12 per cent. In the United States 31 operations have been performed up to March, 1894, with 4 deaths. Analyzing these cases, we find that in not a single one of these fatal cases was the operation elective. Thus: The first fatal case had been in labor twenty-five hours, and was exhausted, with a pulse of 150, when operated upon; the second case died of septic peritonitis; the third died of pneumonia; the fourth had been in labor three days, and died on the eleventh day, of sepsis originating in the subosseous wound.

Of the last 15 operations in the United States there has been 1 death.

In 1893, Pinard, of Paris, performed the operation 13 times. He has had 1 maternal death. She died of sepsis, having been operated upon after she had been in labor three days. The sepsis might have originated before she entered the hospital. Of this last series all the children have been saved. In the last 31 operations in the United States there were 9 foetal deaths. Eight of these children would have been saved had the operation been elective.

From a critical examination of these recent data, it is apparent that the operation of symphysiotomy need not have a mortality rate when it is an elective operation. The sole risk the woman runs is from sepsis,—a risk which is associated with every operation, both major and minor. Here, again, the beneficent doctrine of election comes into the foreground in operative obstetrics.

However bright the prospects of the operation are for the future, it still remains true that for the present it will find its chief field in maternity hospitals. We feel that as yet a sufficient number of cases are not on record to warrant the physician in stating that there are no untoward results as regards locomotion. In private practice, therefore, it is essential, in order to guard against a possible suit for malpractice, to be very guarded in regard to the ultimate prognosis in this respect. Our own feeling in the matter is, that the future will establish this operation on the firm ground of a scientific one, and when that day arrives there will exist no further warrant for the performance of embryotomy on the living in case of the lesser grades of pelvic deformity.

CHAPTER VI. CESAREAN SECTION.

If the foetus is removed from the mother

by means of an incision through the abdominal and uterine walls, the operation is known as Caesarean section. The reader is referred to the numerous monographs which have been written on this subject for its history and the various modifications through which it has passed.

Perhaps of no other operation can it be said that the application of the rules of modern aseptic surgery has accomplished so much as in the one under consideration. It will require time yet, however, before the old prejudice among physicians and laity, engendered by reason of the unnecessary large mortality which accompanied this operation, can be eradicated. Statistics which embrace operations performed ten or even five years ago are of but little value, inasmuch as the technique of the operation has been so modified and perfected that results are entirely different.

The operation now is no longer postponed until the mother's vital forces have been spent in unsuccessful attempts, either on her part or on the part of the obstetrician, in delivering the foetus *per vias naturales. Indications.*—Caesarean section may be performed either from absolute or relative indications. If the pelvic contraction is so marked that delivery of the child by the natural passages be impossible, or if the pelvic canal be obstructed by solid, benign, or malignant growths, the operation is absolutely indicated.

Caesarean section should be performed if the mother is moribund or has just died, if the child is still alive.

The relative indication has a much wider scope, and what is advocated here in this regard would not have been admissible a few years ago, when the mortality rate was so high. However, in the light of recent cases, and when it is remembered how great a mortality exists as a result of embryotomy, and how repulsive it is to every physician to deliberately destroy a life, it is certainly clear that Cesarean section of the future will be done more frequently for relative indications and as an *elective* operation..

Given an instance of pelvic contraction in which the chances are against the delivery of a living child *er vias naiurales,* and the time for induction of premature labor with resulting viable child having elapsed, the obstetrician is justified in performing the Cesarean section, provided always the foetal heart-sounds are clear and regular. The operation is not only done here for relative indications, but is an elective one rather than as a last resort, as has too often been the case. The patient is carefully prepared for it previous to or at the beginning of labor, and, before she has had a chance to become in the least exhausted either by nature or by art, the abdomen is opened and the child delivered. When the operation is considered from this point, embryotomy of the living foetus will become a lost art.

Operation.—Perhaps there is no operation the success of which depends so largely on the many and various little details as in Cesarean section. The operator must have a personal observation of the preparation for the operation, if the best results are to be obtained. Formerly it was thought best to wait for the woman to go into labor before the operation was begun; but in those cases where it has been predetermined that the operation is necessary, it is far better to elect the time of its performance. The old idea that a certain amount of previous cervical dilatation was necessary no longer holds good, in the light of the fact that a few moments only are necessary to sufficiently dilate the cervix. The advantage which is to be gained by the deliberate preparation of the patient, to say nothing of being able to select the hour and light for the operation, more than compensates for the dilatation of the cervix which the normal laborpains would induce. The statement that the uterus will contract more firmly if labor has already begun is purely theoretical, for, in point of fact, experience with just such cases has proven that the uterus does contract firmly as soon as it is emptied.

The operation is much more easily performed if a sufficient number of well-trained assistants are at hand. It is wise, however, that as few hands as possible be introduced into the peritoneal cavity, for, in this way, the possibilities of infection are lessened. There should be an assistant whose sole duty is to administer the anaesthetic; another to assist in lifting out the uterus; another to make compression around the cervix, and still another to assume the charge of the child. Two trained nurses will be necessary to wash sponges and manage the irrigating apparatus. Very few instruments are necessary for this.operation.

Two scalpels, one pair of laparotomy scissors, two dissecting forceps, twelve artery-clamps, four long compressive forceps, one groove-director, one needle-holder, six large and six small curved needles, a Koeberle ecraseur, and a steel dilator should complete the list. A perfectly-new fountain-syringe with a glass tube will answer every purpose as an irrigator. There should be in readiness eighteen sterilized towels.

In place of sponges, pads made of absorbent gauze, large and small, and sterilized, should be used. These should be counted before the operation and just before the abdominal cavity is closed. Five yards of 10-per-cent. iodoform gauze, cut in strips three inches wide and sterilized, should be at hand for intra-uterine tamponade if such prove necessary. A piece of rubber drainage-tubing, three-eighths of an inch in diameter and one yard long, should be boiled and held in readiness in case manual compression should fail to control haemorrhage. Two sizes ol silk (Nos. 4 and 2), silk-worm gut, and some fine catgut should be prepared.

All instruments and ligatures, except catgut, should be boiled immediately preceding the operation and placed in trays containing sterilized water. The operator, his assistants, and nurses must pay special attention to rendering their hands aseptic. Thorough scrubbing with soap and water, washing the hands in alcohol and then a five-minute immersion in 1 to 1000 solution of bichloride of mercury will accomplish this. The operator and his assistants should wear perfectly-clean operating-gowns, or, if these are not at hand, freshly-laundried sheets can be used in their stead. It is the duty of the operator to see that his assistants do not touch anything which has not been rendered aseptic after they have disinfected their hands, without repeating the scrubbing process before they assist in the operation.

Where the operation is one of election and there is time for thorough preparation, the patient should be prepared in the same way as if laparotomy for any other purpose was to be performed. A mild laxative for two or three days previous to the operation should be administered. On the evening previous to the operation the pubic region should be shaved and thoroughly washed. A compress which has been wrung from a solution composed of 1 part of the tincture of green soap and 3 parts of water is placed over the abdomen and held in place by means of an abdominal binder. The next morning the patient is given an enema of soap-suds and a vaginal douche of 1 to 3000 bichloride-of-mercury solution. The towel is removed and the entire surface of the abdomen is washed with 95-per-cent. alcohol and afterward with 1 to 1000 bichloride-of-mercury solution. A piece of damp bichloride gauze should be placed over the abdomen and confined by a few turns of a roller bandage; this the patient should wear to the operating-room. She should be catheterized immediately before the operation.

When the patient is brought to the operating-room she should be placed on a firm table, in the dorsal position with the knees slightly flexed. The upper and lower parts of the body should be covered over with pieces of new rubber cloth, and these in turn be covered with sterilized towels. The abdominal dressing is removed and the abdomen again washed with bichloride-of-mercury solution 1 to 1000. The operator, standing on the patient's right, makes the ordinary laparotomy incision, extending through all the layers of the abdominal wall. This incision can now be safely enlarged, to a point about four inches above the umbilicus, with the scissors, using the fingers of the left hand to protect the intestines. Five or six heavy silk sutures should be passed through the upper three-fourths of the abdominal incision and left untied. The uterus should now be turned out of the abdominal cavity. This is easily accomplished if it is drawn toward the operator so that its left border is made to appear in the wound and then depressing the abdominal wall underneath it. The temporary silk sutures are now to be tightened, care being taken that no loop of intestine is caught within their grasp. The uterus is enveloped in warm sterilized towels and held by the assistant. Sterilised absorbent gauze is placed around the lower segment of the uterus and over the abdominal incision, so that no blood or other fluid may enter the abdominal cavity. A second assistant grasps the lower segment of the uterus with both hands lightly, prepared to control haemorrhage by manual pressure if such become necessary. It is preferred by some to control the uterine bloodsupply by means of a rubber ligature passed around the lower segment of the uterus; but inasmuch as this nearly always causes serious injury to the peritoneum and does not control the haemorrhage any better than can be done manually, it is not advisable.

The uterus is to be opened by making a 4-inch incision through the median line of its anterior surface, embracing the middle third of its length. The assistant who is grasping the lower segment of the uterus should compress it firmly at this time, to control the haemorrhage from the uterine wall.

The incision should be made rapidly, and if the placenta is attached anteriorly it should be pushed to one side and the child extracted. As soon as the child is withdrawn, the assistant whose duty it is to take charge of it should clamp the cord with two compression forceps, cut the cord, and remove the child. The operator at once turns his attention to the placenta, and, if it is adherent, rapidly peels it off. All portions of placental tissue should be carefully removed. It is frequently a wise plan for the assistant whose duty it is to steady the uterus, as soon as the child is extracted, to grasp the edges of the incision between his thumb and fingers, and in this way assist in controlling the haemorrhage from the cut uterine tissue. At this time an hypodermatic injection of the fluid extract of ergot should be made into the gluteal region.

If the cervical canal will easily admit the finger, no dilatation is necessary; otherwise, the steel dilator should be introduced through the incision and the canal gently dilated. The uterus should be packed temporarily with iodoform gauze,—10 per cent.,—and the sutures introduced. The uterine incision should be carefully closed by means of two sets of sutures,—a deep one of No. 2 silk, which passes through all layers of the uterine tissue except the mucous lining, and the sero-serous suture of No. 4 silk.

The deep sutures should enter the uterine tissue one-eighth of an inch from the line of the incision, and, passing diagonally outward into the uterine tissue, re-appear just above the mucous lining of the uterus. The needle used for this suture should be a half-curved, perfectly-round needle, possessing no cutting edge. These sutures should be placed about one-half an inch apart. Time is such an important element in this operation that any device which can safely be used to expedite its performance should be adopted. By threading the needle with a piece of silk sixty inches long, and passing the sutures in the same way as if they were to be continuous, except that the loops be left four or five inches long and afterward cutting all the loops, the sutures can be more rapidly introduced than if each suture is on a separate needle. This is shown in Figs. 61 and 62.

As soon as all the deep sutures are in position, the temporary tamponade in the uterine cavity should be removed and the endometrium sponged out with a weak creolin solution. A 10-per-cent. iodoform-gauze strip, three inches wide and one yard long, is packed into the uterine cavity. One end of the gauze should be carried through the cervical canal into the vagina. This gauze not only provides for freer drainage, but is an additional safeguard against haemorrhage. During the dilatation of the cervical canal and the passage of the gauze strip, the assistant who is controlling the haemorrhage by pressure around the lower uterine segment relaxes his grasp. He should keep up this pressure, except at these times, until the deep sutures are tied.

The sutures which embrace the muscular structure of the uterus are now secured by three knots, after which the ends are cut short.

The sero-serous sutures are of silk also, and interrupted.

Fig. 63. Huture of Uterine Wound. a, deep muscular suture; h, deep muscular suture tied, with the ends rut short; e. Mro-serous lutura passed over deep suture; l. sero-serous suture hetween the deep sutures, ready to be tied.

The Lembert stitch is the ideal one for bringing the peritoneal edges together. The number is almost double that of the deep sutures, one drawing the peritoneum directly over the knot of the deep suture and an intermediate one between each deep suture. The arrangement of both deep and sero-serous sutures is shown in Fig. 63.

As soon as all the sutures have been secured the temporary abdominal sutures are removed and the peritoneal surface of the *cul-de-sac* of Douglas should be sponged out. If any liquor amnii has entered the peritoneal cavity it will be better to sponge it out with Thiersch's solution. When the cavity is sponged dry the abdominal sutures should be introduced.

Silk-worm gut is, perhaps, the best material for this purpose. The abdominal walls are weakened to such an extent by reason of the pregnancy that unusual care must be taken to prevent the occurrence of ventral hernia. Before the suture is passed the assistant should draw the fascia well forward with a pair of mouse-toothed forceps. This suture passes through all layers of the abdominal wall, including the peritoneum. After these sutures are passed the fascia on either side of the incision should be united by means of silk-worm-gut sutures, secured by three knots, and the ends cut short. The deep sutures are now tied, and intermediate approximation sutures used if necessary.

An antiseptic dressing should be placed over the wound and secured by a closely-fitting abdominal binder. If at the conclusion of the operation the patient's pulse is weak and rapid, an enema of whisky and hot salt water should be given before she is removed from the table. The patient should be put to bed and external heat applied to the extremities.

Nothing should be given the patient by mouth during the first twelve hours following the operation except small quantities of hot water to relieve the thirst. If she suffer much pain, she may be given a small dose of morphine hypodermatically. At the end of the first twelve hours, if she has ceased to experience nausea from the ether, small quantities of milk and lime-water can be given, which can gradually be increased according to circumstances.

An attempt should be made to move the patient's bowels as soon as any untoward symptoms, such as a rapid pulse, undue rise of temperature, vomiting, or abdominal distension develop. Otherwise the bowels should not be moved until the third day after the operation.

Calomel triturates, grain each, can be given for this pur pose every hour for six doses. This should be followed by a simple enema.

The patient should receive nothing; but liquid nourishment during the first week after the operation. The ordinary antiseptic pad should be placed over the vulva and renewed as necessary. The intra-uterine drain should be removed on the second or third day. Should the flow at any time be excessive, hypodermatic injections of ergot should be used. Under no circumstances must the patient be allowed to assume the sitting posture during the first ten days.

The abdominal sutures, except those which unite the fascia, should be removed on the tenth day, and with the same care, as regards asepsis, as when they were introduced. The abdominal binder should be worn for one year after the section is performed. Unless some complication prolongs the convalescence, the patient should be up and around her room at the end of three weeks.

This is the method of conducting the elective operation, and, if the patient be in good general condition and the various little details of aseptic surgery are appreciated and executed, the patient should, without any doubt, recover.

If, however, the operation is performed as a last resort, after perhaps thirty or more hours of labor, when the patient's vital forces are greatly lowered from her own and her physician's unsuccessful attempts at delivery, the outlook is by no means so encouraging. On the other hand, the mortality in just such cases is great, as is, in fact, any other operation which may be attempted.

LAPA RO-HYSTERECTOMY.

Before the perfection of the method of performing Cesarean section as it is done to-day, the mortality rate was so high that an attempt was made to eliminate the uterine cavity as a possible source of infection, by removing the uterus after the child had been extracted. This was, without doubt, a great advantage over the old method of either not closing the uterine incision at all or else very imperfectly so.

The operation should not be performed at the present time not only on account of the greater and unnecessary mutilation, but also on account of the increased risk to the patient, unless there be some very well defined indication. If the Caesarean section is performed on a uterus whose endometrium is already the site of sepsis, or if multiple interstitial fibroids complicate the case, or if such marked uterine inertia persist that loss of life from haemorrhage seems imminent, then the entire removal of the uterus is indicated.

Operation—Exactly the same preparations as have been suggested in Caesarean section should be made in case total ablation of the uterus is to be performed, except that a greater number of long compression clamps and a large piece of thin rubber sheeting, such as is used by dentists, should be at hand. The details of the operation are the same as in Caesarean section until the uterus has been turned out of the peritoneal cavity. At this time, instead of using manual compression, a piece of rubber tubing should be passed around the lower uterine segment and loosely tied with one knot. A small opening is now made in the rubber sheeting, which should be made to encircle the uterus just above the rubber tubing. The elasticity of the rubber sheeting will cause it to fit closely around the uterine tissue and prevent any fluid from the uterus entering the peritoneal cavity. With every thing in readiness the assistant draws on the ends of the rubber tubing until the circulation is cut off. The operator at the same time hastily opens the uterus and extracts the child. The placenta is detached and the uterus amputated just above the rubber sheeting with the scalpel. If the endometrium has been the site of septic infection great care must be taken that no fluids enter the peritoneal cavity. The stump above the rubber tubing should be carefully disinfected and seared with the Paquelin cautery. If the patient is in poor condition from either sepsis or other causes, it is better to treat the stump extra-peritoneally, inasmuch as this shortens the operation and lessens shock. If the stump is to be treated extra-peritoneally for the reasons already given, the wire loop of the Koeberle ecraseur should be passed around the stump just below the rubber tubing. It is necessary to see that no portion of the bladder is caught within the grasp of the loop. This accident can be easily prevented if a sound is passed into the bladder to clearly define its attachment to the anterior wall of the cervix. The stump should be firmly compressed with the wire loop until the tissues are blanched. The stump should then be trimmed until it is three-fourths of an inch above the wire. The rubber tubing is removed as soon as the wire is tightened. The stump should again be cauterized and the two pins which accompany the ecraseur passed through the stump, just above the wire, at right angles to the abdominal wound. The peritoneum should now be stitched with catgut around the stump. The *cul-de-sac* of Douglas should be carefully sponged out and the abdominal wall closed.

The operation is completed by powdering the stump with iodoform and applying the usual antiseptic dressings to the abdominal wound. The stump, which of necessity sloughs away, renders the convalescence tedious and the dressings frequent. The stump comes away in ten or twelve days and leaves a granulating surface. If the cervix is now dilated and in this way we permit drainage from below, the wound will heal much more rapidly. A piece of gauze can be passed from above through the cervical canal into the vagina. If, however, the patient's general condition be good, and if the operation is determined upon from an elective stand-point, so that ample preparations can be made, and if the uterine body is the site of multiple fibroids, then the entire uterus, together with the cervix, should be removed. In this case, as soon as the uterus is amputated and the field of operation disinfected, the assistant secures the rubber tubing by tying a double knot. The operator then proceeds to free the bladder from the anterior surface of the lower uterine segment. This can be easily and rapidly done by incising the peritoneum just above the bladder-fold and stripping the bladder-attachment off with the finger. The broad ligament should now be secured on either side by means of very strong silk ligatures. By palpation the uterine artery can be found and secured. The vaginal attachments to the cervix should be cut through and the stump removed. Any bleeding-points should be caught in the forceps and ligated. The ligatures should all be left long, and as soon as all haemorrhage is controlled the ends of the ligatures should be passed into the vaginal opening. Iodoform gauze should be packed in the supravaginal space, and the peritoneum closed by sewing the anterior peritoneal layer of the *cul-de-sac* to the peritoneal covering of the bladder with a continuous catgut ligature. In this way the raw surface is placed entirely extra-peritoneally. The pelvis is carefully sponged and the abdominal wound closed. There is no necessity for drainage from above. The after-treatment should be the same as for Caesarean section.

Laparo-elttrotomy.

The operation for removing the foetus through an incision in the flank possessed advantages at the time when antisepsis and asepsis were unknown, inasmuch as it obviated the necessity of opening the peritoneal cavity. The improved Caesarean section is so much easier of accomplishment, and is fraught with so much less danger, that the necessity for this method no longer exists.

Prognosis.—There is no obstetric operation in which elective surgery plays a greater role in determining the prognosis than the one under consideration. Where the Caesarean section is only determined upon after forceps and version have failed, the woman being exhausted and the child as well, the mortality rate is necessarily high. The elective Caesarean section, on the other hand, so simple and so accurate is its technique, subjects the woman to but one risk, and this is septic infection.

The Caesarean section should alone be judged by its modern fruits. The mortality rate in the past, ranging from 30 to 50 per cent., was due either to faulty technique or to sepsis. At the present, when the advantage of predetermining the operation is recognized, the death-rate, as is noted, barring septic infection, has been lowered approximately to that which is associated with difficult embryotomy.

The latest statistics, as collated by Robert P. Harris, are the following: Of 13 cases where the operation was performed before labor had begun, 10 women recovered and 13 children were saved; of 6 cases where the operation was performed at the beginning of labor, 6 women recovered and 6 children were saved; of 12 cases where the women had been in labor from two to six hours, 10 recovered and 11 children were saved; of 18 cases where the women had been in labor from seven to twelve hours, 8 recovered and 13 children were saved.

These figures speak most eloquently in favor of the elective, predetermined, Caesarean section. Two of the three deaths in the category where the operation was performed before labor had begun were due to septic infection, and the third succumbed to secondary haemorrhage.

The record of individual operators in the United States and abroad surpasses the above statistical data, giving us, in general, a mortality rate varying from *nil* to 10 per cent.

The result of asepsis and of election, then, has been to place the modern Caesarean section on the same plane as other major surgical operations, with the addition of saving from 90 to 95 per cent, of infantile lives otherwise infallibly doomed.

As regards the Porro operation, the prognosis will probably always remain gloomier owing to the extra complications which necessitate resort to it. The mortality rate, however, has been in recent times lowered to about 25 per cent.

CHAPTER VII. EMBRYOTOMY.

Undek the terra "embryotomy" are included a number of operative procedures which have received distinctive names, but the uniform aim of which is to deliver the foetus *per vias iiaturales* after its mutilation to a greater or a less degree. In modern times the sphere of these operations has been greatly narrowed, owing to the perfection in technique and in results of induced labor and of Caesarean section on the one hand, and owing tQ the resuscitation and elevation to a scientific plane of symphysiotomy on the other hand.

Embryotomy, generically considered, includes the following operative procedures: 1. Craniotomy. 2. Cephalotripsy. 3. Evisceration. 4. Decapitation.

In general the indications for these operations are: 1. Contracted pelvis, the foetus being dead or non-viable and the conjugate diameter measuring above two and one-half inches.
2. Obstructed labor, due to monstrosity or to hydrocephalus. 3. Impacted shoulder presentation, impacted after-coming head, or irreducible face presentation, the foetus being dead.

It will be noted that under these indications the proviso is made that the foetus be dead, except when dealing with monstrosities. Our reason for such proviso is the belief, stringently insisted upon throughout this treatise, that, the maternal condition not contra-indicating in the manner sufficiently dwelt upon in the chapters on the Caesarean section and symphysiotomy, recourse to these operations will usually be justifiable, and embryotomy of the live foetus rarely be so. This, at any rate, has become the modern rule in maternity hospitals.

In private practice the question still i-emains open to the choice of the patient, and will so remain until the Caesarean section becomes as safe an operation as, in the hands of an expert, embryotomy should be. In a given case, however, it is the bounden duty of the physician to set the relative standpoints of the two operations impartially before the woman. Neither sentimentality nor religious training or belief should swerve. To speak as definitely as possible, the woman's chances of recovery under embryotomy are fully nine out of ten, but then she loses her child; under the Caesarean section the chances against her are two out of ten, whilst the child's chances of survival are nine out of ten. This fair estimate is, of course, based on the assumption that the Caesarean section is an elective one, and, further,—a point to be well noted,—that the embryotomy of the living foetus is not an elective one, for embryotomy under this condition will never become strictly elective. Where the Caesarean section is not going to be taken into consideration, the average physician, outside of a hospital, will attempt every other possible procedure before deliberately electing an operation which entails the taking of life, even though it be to save life. This is an absolutely erroneous working basis. Where the cause of the pelvic dystocia is recognized, our science is well-nigh exact enough to enable the properly-trained physician to predicate the chance of delivery of the live foetus of average size by means of the non-mutilating minor operations. Therefore, due election is as possible in the case of embryotomy as it is in case of any other obstetric operation. There is no credit in delivering the woman by embryotomy when she is so exhausted as to have but slight chance of surviving the operation. In major dystocia, then, embryotomy of the living foetus should be elected in order to avoid a single percentage of mortality rate; else the maternal chances from the Caesarean section are far better than from non-elective embryotomy. That is to say, where the choice between the two operations is based on an absolute indication, the one or the other must be deliberately elected. It is the border-line cases which will always call for the soundest judgment, and here, fortunately, symphysiotomy can stand between the Caesarean section and embryotomy of the living foetus. As is amply emphasized under the subject of symphysiotomy, there is to-day left little ground for the choice of embryotomy. Under an absolute indication the Caesarean section is as safe for the woman as the difficult embryotomy, and under the relative indication pubic section narrows very strictly the indications of embryotomy. In the near future, then, the physician in private practice, as he is now in hospital practice, may be relieved of the duty of killing the foetus in cases where, through an alternate operation, both woman and foetus may be saved.

1. *The Operation of Craniotomy.*—This operation, as the name implies, aims at diminishing the bulk of the foetal skull. It is performed either on the beforecoming or on the altercoming head. In the latter event it will rarely become a question of killing the foetus, since the child will usually be dead before craniotomy is demanded. At best, craniotomy must be considered a difficult operation. The working room is slight owing to the contraction of the pelvis; for the same reason the cervix is rarely fully dilated; injury to the maternal parts is not an unlikely occurrence, and this traumatism increases greatly the risk from septic infection or, in any event, will complicate the convalescence.

The essential instruments requisite for the performance of craniotomy are: A trephine for perforation; a cranioclast for extraction. There are a number of types of perforators, such as Karl Braun's trephine, Blot's perforator,

Martin's trephine, Naegele's scissors. Braun's and Blot's instruments are particularly useful in case the operation is performed on the beforecoming head; the scissors answers best for the aftercoming head.

The head having been perforated, a sound (like the uterine or, better still, the metal urethral) is needed to break up the

Fig. 67.—Scissors-Perforator.

brain, and a syringe to wash out the contents of the cranium. This accomplished, the cranioclast or craniotractor—a better term, since it defines the purpose of the instrument—comes into play. The best instrument is that of Karl Braun.

The steps of the operation are the following: The external genitals and the vagina having been thoroughly asepticized, the woman is placed on a table, the bed not sufficing for any of the major obstetric operations. The instruments are sterilized and the hands of the operator and of his assistant are carefully cleansed. Too much care in this respect is not possible, since the sole risk in expert hands to which the woman is subjected is septic infection. If the woman be not excessively nervous, and the operative indication be not an extreme one, anaesthesia is not absolutely essential. In view, however, of its safety, we always counsel it.

The bladder having been emptied by catheter, the woman is placed in the lithotomy position and we proceed as follows:— (a) *Craniotomy of the Before-coming Head.*—The foetal head should be steadied at the brim through supra-pubic pressure made by an assistant. The operator determines the position of the head through vaginal examination and selects the preferable point for perforation. Either a parietal or the occipital bone will be accessible, and one or the other should be chosen, sutures and fontanelles being avoided. The ringers of the left hand are placed against the foetal head to steady the trephine and to guard against injury to the maternal parts. The trephine is pressed firmly against the head, its handle is steadied by the operator's right hand, and the nurse or the second assistant turns the screw of the trephine until the head has been entered. The trephine is now removed and the metal sound is inserted into the cranium to break up the brain. The nozzle of the syringe or a glass irrigating tube, fitted to. the syringe, next takes the place of the sound and the brain is washed out. (Plate XIV, Fig. 1.)

It has been contended that the preferable practice is now to leave the case to nature. We can see no advantage in this. The woman being anaesthetized, it is better to follow perforation with extraction. We thus avoid what may prove futile efforts on nature's part, and we thus forestall possible maternal exhaustion. The left or grooved blade of Braun's cranioclast is inserted into the opening made by the trephine; the other blade is applied to the outside of the skull, being guided into position by fingers of the right or left hand, according as the blade is applied to the left or the right of the pelvis. The blades are locked; the screw is turned home, which results in firm hold of the head being secured. Traction is made, even as with the forceps, in the axis of the pelvic brim until the head reaches the pelvic floor, and then in the axis of the pelvic outlet. The foetus having been extracted and the placenta having been expressed, an intra-uterine douche of 2-per-cent. creolin or of 1 to 8000 bichloride solution is given.

Fig. 69.—Etfect of the Cranioclast on the Foetal Skull.

Where extraction by the cranioclast proves difficult owing to non-yielding of the occiput, the cephalotribe, as will be noted, should be substituted. It is to be remembered that extraction by the cranioclast is possible because, the cranial contents having been evacuated, traction on the head causes it to be compressed, and thereby diminished by the pressure exerted by the pelvic walls Undue pressure is to be avoided in order to prevent, in turn, traumatism of the maternal parts.

(b) *Craniotomy of the After-coming Head.*—The operation on the after-coming head presents greater difficulties than that on the before-coming head. The trunk of the foetus having been extracted, it is in the way of the necessary manipulations. Only exceptionally, also, will it be possible to elect the desirable point for perforation, this point being the occipitoatloid ligament. Further still, after perforation and excerebration, if the head be wedged tightly at the brim, the greatest possible care is requisite, in inserting the blades of the extractor, in order to avoid inflicting considerable traumatism on the maternal parts.

When possible to reach the occipito-atloid ligament, the scissors-perforator of Naegele is the best instrument. When the necessities of the case require perforation through the dense mastoid or occipital bone, the perforator of Martin or of Blot, being smaller than the trephine of Braun, should be selected.

The steps of the operation are as follow: After thorough asepsis of the genital tract and emptying of the bladder, one assistant steadies the head by supra-pubic pressure, and a second pulls the trunk of the foetus laterally, downward or upward, according as the operator has decided to perforate under the pubes, to one or the other side of the pelvis, or from below upward. If the occiput has been rotated under the pubes, as it ordinarily may, the operator determines with the finger the occipito-atloid articulation, and guides the scissors along this finger to the site. The finger must remain in position during perforation, in order to protect the bladder in the event of the scissors slipping. The wedge of the scissors having been entered at the articnlation. pressure on the handles enlarges the opening into the cranium laterally, and next, by rotation of the scissors, similar pressure enlarges the opening antero-posteriorly. This having been effected, the scissors is removed and the metal sound is inserted for the purpose of breaking up the brain. The contents of the cranium are next washed out with sterilized water thrown in by the syringe. If the pelvic contraction be not marked and uterine contractions are active, the excerebrated head may be bom spontaneously. As a rule, however, extraction by the cranioclast is essential. The left, grooved blade of Braun's cranioclast is inserted into the cranial cavity, the right blade is applied laterally, the instrument is locked, and the screw is turned home. Traction is made in the axis of the pelvic inlet or outlet, according to whether the head is in the cavity or on the pelvic floor. (Plate XIV, Fig. 2.)

If the position of the head is such that the occipito-atloid ligament cannot be reached, it becomes necessary to enter the skull through an opening made in one or another of the cranial bones, and then the scissors-perforator will not answer. Either Blot's or Martin's instrument is firmly applied to the point selected for perforation, and the skull is trephined. The other steps are similar to those just stated.

At times the foetal head is extended at the outlet, so that practically we are dealing with an impacted face presentation. Under these circumstances the skull may be entered with the scissors-perforator through the roof of the mouth.

Exceptionally, owing to density of the cranium, it becomes impossible to extract with the cranioclast. Then, as will be noted, it becomes necessary to resort to cephalotripsy.

The operation of craniotomy having been completed and the placenta having been expressed, an intra-uterine douche of 2-per-cent. creolin or of 1 to 8000 bichloride solution should be administered. In the event of injury having been inflicted on the pelvic floor, the same should be repaired.

2. *The Operation of CephalotHpsy.*—The aim of this operation is to crush the skull in order to allow of readier extraction than is possible in certain instances by means of the cranioclast. The latter instrument is a tractor, pure and simple; the cephalotribe is at the outset a crusher and afterward a tractor. Perforation is as essential an initial step as in a case of craniotomy. The advantage, therefore, which the cephalotribe has over the cranioclast is that, being a more powerful instrument, it enables the operator to overcome the difficulties in the way of delivery by the simple tractor offered by a dense and fully-ossified cranium. The cephalotribe, however, has the disadvantage of being a bulkier instrument than the cranioclast, and, further, occupies more space in the pelvis, since neither of the blades is applied within the cranial cavity. For this reason, therefore, the cranioclast is to be preferred whenever the emergencies of the given case will allow of its application.

Simpson, Hicks, Breisky, Lusk, and others have devised useful forms of the instrument. Lusk's cephalotribe, in most respects, will answer best where the instrument is indicated at all. Obviously, since the cephalotribe is applied entirely between the walls of the pelvis and the foetal head, and since, further, the instrument, whilst diminishing the diameter of the head in one direction, increases it in another, is applicable only when the operation is indicated in the presence of the minor grades of pelvic contraction.

Exceptionally, even this instrument is not powerful enough to break up the base of the cranium to permit of delivery without subjecting the maternal parts to unnecessary damage. Then we must have recourse to the rather complicated, but most powerful, instrument devised by Tarnier,—the basiotribe. This instrument is a perforator and a cephalotribe in one. The screw-tip perforates the cranium and holds it firmly whilst the action of the blades is crushing the base of the skull.

Notwithstanding its advantages in certain cases, the cephalotribe is a more dangerous instrument than the cranioclast. Injury to the maternal parts is more likely owing to the increased room in the pelvis its use entails; and, further, owing to the spicula of bone which are apt to project as the result of the crushing force applied. Still, the instrument is a most essential one in fortunately rare instances.

The initial steps of cephalotripsy are similar to those for craniotomy,—thorough asepsis of the genital tract, hands of operator and assistant and instruments, followed by perforation and excerebration. The blades of the cephalotribe are next applied accurately to the foetal head, under the guidance of the fingers in the vagina. The screw is then turned home and the cranium is crushed, being elongated in the diameter opposed to to that in which the crushing force is exerted. This latter point is ever to be borne in mind, so that during the process of extraction the enlarged diameter of the foetal skull may be rotated, where choice exists, into the larger diameter of the pelvis. Extraction is made even as with the forceps, in the axis of the inlet, until the head reaches the pelvic floor, and then in the axis of the outlet. After delivery of the foetus and the placenta, an intra-uterine douche of 2-per-cent. crcolin or 1 to 8000 bichloride solution is to be administered, and any injury to the pelvic floor is to be repaired.

3 and 4. *Evisceration and Decapitation.*—These operations are applicable to instances where the foetus lies transversely in the uterus, and impacted to such a degree as to forbid version, for the purpose of bringing the foctal head in such relation to the pelvic brim as to permit of craniotomy.

Evisceration is called for where the neck of the foetus cannot be reached, whereas, when it can be reached, decapitation finds its sphere of action. Both these operative procedures must be considered as well-nigh the most dangerous of all obstetric operations. Aside from the increased risk of direct traumatism to the uterus, in which organ, necessarily, the manipulations take place, the lower uterine segment is usually thinned, particularly in neglected cases, and, therefore, there exists considerable likelihood of rupture of the uterus.

Where the neck of the uterus is not accessible and evisceration becomes the operation of necessity, the steps are as follow: After thorough asepsis of the genital tract, and similar precautions in regard to the hands of the operator, his assistants, and the requisite instruments, the scissors-perforator is guided along one or more fingers in the vagina to the most accessible portion of the foetal trunk, is inserted to its full depth, and the opening thus made is enlarged by pressure on the handles. The metallic sound is next inserted into this opening, and the contained organs are broken up. This process is tedious and calls for extreme caution lest the sound perforate the foetus, and thus inflict damage on the uterus. Whenever possible the finger of the operator should take the place of the sound. The cavity having been emptied of its contents, any projecting spiculaa of bone are removed by the bone-forceps, and then the foetal trunk may possibly be bent on itself through traction applied by the blunt hook, and be thus delivered. Should this manipulation fail, the operator will be obliged to break the foetus up further, dismembering it, and resorting to the cranioclast or to the cephalotribe for the extraction of the foctal head. A number of complicated instruments, such as chain-saws, have been devised for use in these extreme instances; but they are one and all open to the objection that, being difficult to apply around the foetal trunk, they are liable to inflict great damage on the maternal structures. A simple device is the following: When possible a sterilized gum-elastic catheter, threaded through its eye with a stout sterilized cord, is carried around the trunk of the foetus. The catheter is unthreaded and removed, leaving the cord around the foetus. The ends of this cord are brought out of the vagina through a cylindrical speculum, and then, by traction on the ends of the cord, the foetal trunk may usually be sawn through. This failing, the sole alternative is to cut through the spinal column by the scissors. The name of *spondylotomy* has been applied to these procedures. Such an amount of traumatism is thus entailed that we question if, where the conjugate is diminished below two and three-fourths inches, it be not preferable to enlarge the pelvic diameters by symphysiotomy in order to obtain greater working space.

Where the neck of the foetus is accessible decapitation is the operation of choice. A number of instruments, complicated to a greater or less degree, have been devised for the performance of decapitation. The simplest of all is the Braun hook or *decollator*. This hook can be used in every instance where the more complicated apparatus can; it is serviceable where the latter is not, for the reason that if there is not space enough to pass the decollator it is likewise impossible to adapt the chain-saw; it is readily rendered aseptic and is less likely to injure the maternal parts than any of the other devices.

In an emergency, where the Braun instrument is not at hand, a stout sterilized cord may be carried around the foetal neck by means of a sterilized elastic catheter; the ends of the cord are carried through a cylindrical speculum out of the vagina, and a see-saw motion associated with traction will sever the head from the trunk. Whenever possible, however, the Braun hook is to be preferred, and the steps of the operation are as follow: The bladder is to be emptied. The genital tract, the hands of the operator and of his assistants having been carefully asepticized, the foetal arm is brought down out of the 7

Fig. 71.—Braun's Hook or Decollator.

vagina and handed to an assistant, who, through the exerted traction, steadies the foetal neck at the brim and makes it more accessible. It is desirable to exert traction on this arm by means of a tape or towel tied to it, otherwise the assistant will be in the way of the operator.

The aim of the operator is to pass the hook around the neck of the foetus, and this is accomplished as follows: Inserting two fingers of the right or the left hand (according as the foetal head occupies the left or the right half of the pelvis) into the vagina, the hook is passed flat along these fingers until the neck of the foetus is reached. The point of the hook is then guided around the neck by these fingers from above downward, in order to lessen the risk of injuring the bladder. (Plate XV.)

Firm traction is then made on the hook in order to assure a thorough hold on the neck, the fingers remaining in place so as to certify that the point of the hook is not injuring the maternal parts. The hook is rotated, traction being maintained until the neck is felt to yield through the breaking of the spinal column. As a rule, the soft parts also are thus severed, and the hook is removed along the fingers. If the hook has failed to sever completely the muscular attachments, the scissors, guided along the fingers, must be utilized.

The neck of the foetus having been severed, traction on the prolapsed fcetal arm will ordinarily serve to deliver the trunk, the foetal head slipping upward. The next step is to remove the head.

If the indication for decapitation has been an impacted transverse position of the dead foetus, in a pelvis where there exists no special disproportion between the pelvis and the fcetus, the forceps will answer for extraction. The head being steadied at the pelvic brim by an assistant, the forceps is applied in the usual manner, and delivery is effected under the rules applicable to the forceps operation.

Where, however, there exists dystocia due to contracted pelvis or to large fcetus, the manipulations become more difficult according to the degree of dystocia. The method of inserting the blunt hook into the cranium through the foramen magnum and delivering by traction has been advocated, but should be rejected owing to the risk of the hook slipping and injuring the maternal parts. The preferable method is the following:

If the head can be fixed at the brim with the foramen magnum presenting toward the vagina, then excerebration by the metal sound and extraction by the cranioclast or the cephalotribe is advisable. If the head cannot be so fixed, then perforation by the trephine or the scissors-perforator is demanded, followed by extraction by the cranioclast or the cephalotribe. The risk to the maternal parts is here great, owing to the fact that the point of impact of the trephine or scissors can rarely be at a right angle, and there is, therefore, great danger of the instruments slipping. If the pelvis be large enough to permit of its introduction, Tarnier's basiotribe will answer admirably.

The uterus having been emptied, a 2-per-cent. creolin or a 1 to 81)00 bichloride douche should be administered, and lesion of the genital tract be repaired as completely as is possible.

Aside from impacted transverse presentation, decapitation may be called for in case of locked twins.

The trunk of one foetus having been born, and it being found impossible by manual and postural treatment to decompose the wedge formed by the foetal heads, the only possible resource is the sacrificing of the first foetus—in case it be not already dead—in order to give the second foetus chance of life; for it is the first foetus, the trunk of which is born, whose life is most endangered. The steps of the operation do not differ from those just stated.

Prognosis Of Embryotomy.

It is not possible to state specifically the death-rate from embryotomy. The statistical data at disposal are worthless, because of the fact that many of the records include operations performed before the stringency of asepsis was recognized, and, further, because the operation, except under absolute indication, has rarely been one of election. It is a significant fact that the mortality following embryotomy is higher in private than in hospital practice. The reason is that in the former practice the temptation is to test the methods of delivery by forceps and version before resorting to embryotomy; often because accurate mensuration of the pelvis having been neglected, the practitioner is unawaie of the cause of the dystocia till his eyes are opened by the fact that the methods of delivery with which he is most familiar are of no avail. Embryotomy is then resorted to on an exhausted woman with genital tract already damaged, to a greater or less degree, by the futile efforts at delivery by methods which the mechanical problem forbid. Deliberate election of embryotomy, on the other hand, is more likely to be the rule in hospitals, and, therefore, the mortality is lower. Further still, the mortality depends on the indication for the operation selected. Where the dystocia is not extreme and the operation, therefore, not a difficult one, the sole risk entailed by embryotomy is sepsis. In the higher degrees of dystocia, particularly where evisceration is called-for, the mortality must always remain relatively high owing to the lesions which, even in the hands of the most expert, the maternal parts are likely to incur.

Minor lesions, such as lacerations of the cervix or of the pelvic floor, if repaired at once and aseptically, are not likely to enter as complications of the puerperal state. Neither are fistulae, if the result of direct traumatism and not of sloughing following prolonged pressure. The major risk the woman runs is rupture of the uterus,—a not unlikely accident where embryotomy is demanded in a justo-minor pelvis of high grade through an undilated cervix. Whilst, indeed, embryotomy may prove a very simple operation, it may also become the most difficult of all the obstetric operations. For this reason, when the child is alive, it has become the custom in hospitals to weigh carefully the chances in the boundary-line cases of Caesarean section and of embryotomy. It becomes a question not, as is often erroneously argued, of the greater value of one life over another; it becomes a question of the deliberate, scientific election of that operation which subjects the woman to the least risk. There is no doubt but that difficult embryotomy, in the hands of the non-expert, subjects the woman to greater risk than does the Cesarean section, provided always that he is familiar with the simple technique of the latter operation, as he should be, if competent to attend the lying-in woman at all.

CHAPTER VIII. THE SURGERY OF THE PUERPERITJM.

The puerperal state begins with the expulsion of the placenta, which event terminates the third stage of labor. In case surgical interference has been required during the course of labor, the genital tract has likely enough suffered certain lesions which it becomes the duty of the physician to repair. As a rule, the surgery requisite may be denominated minor, with the exception of one complication,—rupture of the uterus.

In the event of the labor or the surgical interference not having been conducted aseptically, there will develop, during the course of the puerperal state, a number of complications, which may also require surgical intervention, and, as a rule, this surgery is of a major nature.

The operations, then, which we are called upon to consider depend either on traumatism, avoidable or unavoidable, or on sepsis, which, from the modern stand-point, must be looked upon as almost always avoidable.

The operations resulting from traumatism are the following: 1. Laceration of the cervix. 2. Laceration of the pelvic floor. 3. Fistuhe. 4. Rupture of the uterus.

The affections depending on septic infection which may demand surgical interference are: 1. Endometritis and metritis. 2. Pelvic abscess. 3. Peritonitis. 4. Mastitis.

Immediate Repair Of The Lacerated Cervix.

It is only of late years that it has been considered desirable to attempt the immediate repair of the lacerated cervix. The objections to the operation have been the problematical result as regards primary union and, further, the belief that it was impossible to resort to the operation without the presence of a number of assistants. There are now a sufficient number of cases recorded to warrant the assertion that primary nnion may usually be expected, and if the technique we proceed to describe be followed skilled assistants are not necessary. On the other hand, the primary operation shuts off one of the avenues of sepsis, and removes at once one of the most frequent causes of subinvolution, as well as, in case of union, relieves the patient of the necessity of the secondary operation.

The immediate operation is either one of election or one of strict necessity. It becomes one of necessity when, either after spontaneous labor or after operative interference, profuse haemorrhage occurs and continues, which, on investigation, is found to be due to a cervical tear involving a circular artery. Here the only other resource is tamponing the vagina, which is unscientific as well as often nugatory. The operation becomes one of election in the lesser degrees of laceration. Unquestionably many such lacerations heal spontaneously, probably the vast majority if the course of the puerperium is aseptic. Still, we question if, where the laceration exceeds what may be termed the first degree, the patient has not the right to expect her physician to leave her in the best possible condition, in order to save her from the grasp of the gynaecologist later.

In case the operation is called for on account of laceration involving the circular artery, there exists no contra-indication. The immediate safety of the woman demands it. There are contraindications to the performance of the operation in the presence of the lesser grades of laceration. If the woman is exhausted from prolonged labor, or if, owing to post-partum haemorrhage, it has become necessary to use the uterine tamponade, then resort to the operation is either inadvisable or impracticable.

The instruments requisite for the performance of the operation arc the following: A strong vulsellum forceps, a needle-holder, and a few large curved needles, preferably the Hagedorn. The preferable suture material is silk-worm gut. Catgut is unreliable, since it is apt to dissolve too soon and, furthermore, because the knot is apt to slip. The silkworm gut is readily sterilized by boiling for a few minutes, and may be left *in situ* for weeks, as may be requisite, if, at the same time, it is necessary to repair the pelvic floor. A speculum is not strictly requisite, since, according to the technique about to be described, the operation is performed without one. The main advantage in dispensing with a speculum is that thus an assistrant to hold it is not required. If the operator happen to have an Edebohl speculum with him, however, the counter-weight may be obtained by means of a flat-iron, which is to be found in every household.

The steps of the operation are the following: The woman is brought to the edge of the bed; the bladder is emptied; anaesthesia is only requisite in case the woman is excessively nervous. If the requisite assistants—two in number— are present, each may support a leg; but, in the event of these assistants not being present, the physician may use a sheet as a leg-holder by passing it around the knees and tying it to the patient's arms. The requisite instruments, having been sterilized by boiling, are placed handy to the operator's right hand, a lighted candle or lamp, in case the gaslight is not sufficient, being held by the nurse or by some relative so as to illuminate the field of operation thoroughly.

The operator seizes the cervical lips firmly with the double tenaculum, and pulls the uterus downward until the cervix is at the ostium vaginae. The object of this traction is twofold: In the first place, the laceration is thus made accessible for operation, being performed under the guidance of the eye, and, in the second place, when the uterus is thus pulled downward, it is a well-known fact that haemorrhage from the organ is, in a measure, checked. For this reason the technique described is preferable to that which entails operating through the Sims speculum, when the haemorrhagic flow which always exists after the completion of labor renders the operation difficult by interfering with the field of vision. The next step is to pass the first and the most difficult of the stitches, which, once in place, gives the operator lull control. A Hagedorn needle threaded with silkworm gut is passed deeply, at the angle through the posterior cervical lip, under the lacerated surface, emerging in the canal. It is re-inserted into the anterior lip at the canal, and emerges at the angle of the tear in the anterior lip. The remaining stitches are inserted in a similar manner, first on the one side, and next on the other, until the raw surfaces of each lip have been approximated. The sutures are

Fig. 77.—Sutures Inserted on One Side of a Lacerated Cervix.

next tied. It is important to remember that it is essential to tie the stitches tighter after the primary operation than after the secondary, when the aim is simply to bring the denuded surfaces in apposition. After delivery, the cervix is always oedematous to a greater or less degree, and, if the stitches be not tied tightly then, in the course of a few days, when the oedema disappears, the stitches will necessarily be slack and deep union by first intention is unlikely. It is to the neglect of this precaution, we believe, that failure after the primary operation may often be traced.

The sutures having been tied, the vulsellum forceps is removed and a hot 2-per-cent. creolin douche is administered. The average time requisite lor this operation is ten minutes. In case of failure in obtaining union, the woman's condition is none the worse for the attempt made to leave her in the best possible condition, whilst, as already stated, if union do occur, the woman is spared many of the ills which a lacerated cervix sooner or later entails. There is a further phase of this question which it is well to dwell upon. If the immediate operation be not performed in case of deep cervical laceration, dense cicatricial tissue inevitably forms, so that when the secondary operation is called for there is not alone much more difficulty in performance, but it may even, in the opinion of many, become not a question of mere repair of a laceration, but one of amputation,—a more radical operation. We believe that before long it will be recognized as desirable to perform immediate trachelorrhaphy, as it is to-day considered a sign of incompetency if repair of the pelvic floor is not attended to immediately, in the absence of contra-indication.

The stitches in the cervix may be left *in situ* from ten days to a number of weeks, according to the necessities of the case. The longer interval is requisite where it has also been necessary to operate on the pelvic floor. If the stitches are aseptic, as they should be, when introduced, they can give rise to no possible trouble during the puerperal state. The assumption that they may interfere with drainage of the lochia is untenable, since the operation simply restores the cervix to the shape it has where laceration has not occurred. It goes without saying that we presuppose that requisite care has been taken not to sew up the cervical canal.

Immediate Perineorrhaphy.

The conscientious physician aims to leave his patient, after confinement, with the pelvic floor in as sound a condition as art can make it, in the event of its having been lacerated during the process of delivery. There is little need at the present day to dwell on the untoward sequelae which inevitably follow in the train of unrepaired lesion of the pelvic floor. The laity, as well as physicians in general, recognize the necessity of the primary operation,—so much so, indeed, that the former consider their medical attendant blameworthy who has failed to recognize a lesion, and thus neglected to repair it. The student need not have the fear that, if the lesion occur, it will be laid to his lack of skill. The practitioner who claims that, in an extensive practice, he has never seen a lacerated perineum has become to-day a *vara avis* in the light of the recorded experience from hospitals which certify to the necessarily frequent occurrence of lesion even in the hands of the most expert. The proper spirit to-day is to fear the blame which deservedly attaches itself to the attendant who neglects the performance of the primary operation whenever the conditions contra-indicating are absent.

The routine practice, after the completion of the third stage of labor, shoidd be to investigate by sight, as well as by touch, the pelvic floor. There may be no apparent lesion externally, and yet, on separation of the labia, the most dangerous of all lesions, as regards its after-consequences, will be detected. It is now firmly established that the mere external tears are of no consequence beyond opening an avenue for the entrance of germs. It is the tears which involve the muscles and fascia of the pelvic floor which entail ultimately rectocele and cystocele, with their sequela?. Too much stress, therefore, cannot be laid on the necessity of separating the labia and examining the pelvic floor.

The sole contra-indication to the immediate operation is exhaustion of the woman to such a degree, from prolonged labor or from post-partum haemorrhage, as to call for absolute and immediate rest on her part. Of course, where, owing to post-partum luemorrhage, it has been necessary to resort to the gauze tamponade of the genital tract, the operation canuot be performed. Where the lesion, at best, requires but a few stitches, anaesthesia is not requisite, since the sensibility of the pelvic floor has been largely diminished from the pressure associated with delivery. But, if the tear be one of a major degree, anaesthesia is desirable in order to enable the attendant to perform the operation with the requisite care as well as in order to save the woman unnecessary pain.

The instruments requisite are the following: A pair of scissors, a needle-holder, a few curved needles (preferablv the Hagedorn). Material for suture will differ according to individual preference, but the silk-worm gut possesses all the advantages of silver wire or catgut, and has none of the disadvantages of the latter. Where the tear is chiefly internal, catgut, if its asepticism can be depended upon, answers admirably, since it is possible to use it as a running suture; but even then it may dissolve before deep union is secured, or, notwithstanding the precautions taken, it may prove the source of local sepsis. As for silver wire, it possesses no advantages for the primary operation over silk-worm gut, and requires infinitely more time for adjustment as well as more instruments. Silk-worm gut is readily sterilized by boiling, and, if aseptic, it may be left *in situ* for an indefinite time.

The method of operating will be modified according to the character of the laceration. The most complex operation, of course, is demanded where the laceration extends through the sphincter ani, to a greater or a less extent, up the rectal wall. In the lesser grades the suturing usually will be almost entirely within the vagina. Before proceeding to operate the physician should make a careful examination in order to determine the manner after which the pelvic floor has been injured, in order to secure deep union and proper approximation of the fascia and muscles. The ancient method of simply passing the sutures in at one side and out at the other will not stand the critical test of modern methods, for the day has gone by when securing a skin perineum is deemed sufficient. The parts operated upon must not alone look well, but must also subserve their intended purpose well.

Where the laceration has not extended through the sphincter of the anus the steps of the operation are as follow: The woman is brought to the edge of the bed, the legs are flexed on the abdomen and are held there by the nurse, or, if she is needed for other purposes, a sheet may be passed under the knees and each end tied to the patient's arms. As a rule, except in the minor degrees of laceration, anaesthesia is requisite. In order to avoid sponging, the field of operation may be irrigated to advantage by a weak solution of bichloride. Creolin is objectionable for irrigating purposes, since, owing to its color, it interferes with a good view of the field of operation. An assistant or the nurse, with aseptic hands, separates the labia so that the operator may determine the extent of the laceration. With the scissors jagged ends of tissue are cut off, thus securing an even surface for union. If the laceration has extended chiefly into one sulcus, as is not infrequently the case in the lesser degrees of lesion, a running catgut suture may be used to advantage. The needle is inserted at the apex of the tear, deeply, so as to secure as much of the divided fascia as possible, and the gut is tied. The over-and-over stitch is now rapidly taken, the needle on each occasion it is inserted being made to enter deeply, until the external end of the laceration has been reached, when it is tied. Occasionally the tear involves both sulci, in which event the process is repeated on the other side. In order to see well, the upper vagina is tamponed with sterilized gauze, which prevents the trickling of the uterine discharges.

In general, however, Hegar's method of operating (modified) will give the most satisfactory result, even though its performance takes more time than that which we have just described.

The method is peculiarly applicable to the vast majority of lacerations, since these begin in the median line and extend laterally. The suturing is almost entirely internal, and approximates accurately the divided ends of the muscles and fascia, the aim which is essential in order to properly repair the lesion.

The needle is inserted at the margin of the tear near its apex, and passed deeply around to the opposite side. Similar sutures are inserted at an interval of about a quarter of an inch apart, till the tear has been approximated down to the carunculae myrtiformes. The sutures are then tied and cut short. The superficial tear remaining is brought together by two or more sutures. Silk-worm gut answers admirably, and, if need be, a few interrupted sutures of catgut may be inserted. These sutures, if aseptic, may remain in place for a week or ten days. If there exist much oedema of the pelvic floor, the result of protracted labor, the precaution must be taken to tie the sutures a trifle tighter than is the rule for plastic work; otherwise, on the disappearance of the oedema, the sutures will be relaxed and deep union will not be secured.

Where the laceration has been so extensive as to involve not only the pelvic floor, but also the sphincter ani and the recto-vaginal septum, there is all the more call for the immediate operation, and the procedure is proportionately more complicated. It is above all things important to bring together the torn ends of the sphincter ani, for otherwise the woman will suffer from incontinence of faeces to a greater or less degree, and will, in consequence, inevitably require the secondary operation. In this operation we still prefer the silk-worm gut for suture

Fig. 79.—Laceration through the Sphincter. Sphincter Sutures in Place. purposes. It holds just as well as silver wire, and is a source of less discomfort to the woman. The first stitches to be inserted are the rectal. The needle is inserted below the margin of the tear and is carried deeply outward so as to grasp the torn ends of the sphincter. It circles around the recto-vaginal septum and emerges at the opposite side, grasping the other end of the sphincter. As a rule, two sutures are requisite to secure the sphincter muscle, and when inserted these may be tied. The laceration of the pelvic floor is then repaired according to the method just described.

Exceptionally, the laceration occurs directly through the perineum, giving rise to what is termed central laceration. In case of this accident, the method of procedure consists in converting the central laceration into a complete, by slitting through the bridge of tissue remaining between the laceration and the pelvic floor, and then repairing the lesion after the method described.

If the steps of the operations just described are aseptic, the management of the puerperal state does not differ materially from the normal. It is unnecessary to administer vaginal douches, since the non-septic lochia will not interfere with union. The old-time rule of keeping the bowels constipated is not deemed good practice to-day. The comfort of the puerpera demands that the intestinal canal should not be allowed to become clogged, and the perineal tear is more likely to heal from the depths if we take precautions to prevent hardened faecal matter from collecting in the rectal *cul-de-sac*. It is a good rule, therefore, to order a saline laxative within twenty-four hours after delivery, and thereafter every day, so as to secure copious liquid evacuations. The coaptated surface may be kept powdered with iodoform, aristol, or boracic acid, and the nurse should be strictly enjoined to exercise scrupulous cleanliness of the external genitals. For the first few days the woman had better be catheterized, or else, and this we prefer, when she passes water it should be under the administration of a weak creolin or bichloride douche. It is very questionable if the normal urine will interfere at all with primary union.

In the event of the primary operation proving a failure, the woman should be advised to submit to the secondary operation as early as may be, for the longer she waits the greater the cicatricial tissue, and the more aggravated the rectocele and possibly the cystocele which will form.

Fistula.

Only exceptionally, nowadays, are fistulae of the genital tract encountered, for the reason that their chief causes are not allowed to act. Protracted labor was formerly responsible for the majority of fistulae. Traumatism, except in the presence of a major degree of pelvic contraction when surgical interference was demanded, was rarely a causative factor. It is only when a fistula forms as the result of surgical interference that the physician, in the capacity of accoucheur, will be called upon to perform immediate operation. The fistulae which result from prolonged pressure of the fœtal presenting part on the pelvic floor rarely make themselves evident until a number of days after labor. The process is purely one of sloughing in these latter instances. Of course, here, as well, it is eminently necessary to take measures for repair of the lesion as soon as the condition of the woman will allow, since the formation of extensive cicatrices will render the operation most difficult and the result problematical.

In view of the difficulty of the secondary operation for fistula, it may at first sight seem useless to attempt repair immediately after delivery. When we remember, however, the untoward sequelae of both urinary and finecal fistulas, and the repeated attempts which are often requisite before union can be secured after the secondary operation, there is little need of dwelling further on the desirability of aiming at primary union. The main reason why the primary operation is difficult is the impossibility of placing the recently delivered puerpera in the best position for performing the operation, particularly when the fistula affects the bladder. This, indeed, will prove a distinct contra-indication when the fistula is seated high up; but when the lesion is low enough down to enable the physician to bring it into view without placing the woman in the genu-pectoral position, the attempt at primary repair should always be made, liectal fistula? may ordinarily be exposed with less difficulty than the vesical.

The steps of the operation either for rectal or vesical fistula? do not differ from those requisite for the performance of the secondary operation. To prevent the lochia from trickling down and interfering with the field of vision, it suffices to pack the upper portion of the vagina with sterilized gauze. Since there is no cicatricial tissue and, consequently, no special tension to be overcome, silk-worm gut will answer for suture purposes.

If the fistula is at all accessible with the woman in the dorsal position, the edges are made tense by traction with a tenaculum, and the sutures are inserted one after another from one edge of the fistula out at the other. The same care is requisite, as in the secondary operation, not to pass the stitches through the vesical wall. Coaptation of the torn edges must be accurate and the stitches must be tied more tightly than in the secondary operation, because when any oedema present has disappeared the stitches will otherwise become relaxed.

The after-treatment will not differ from that of the normal puerperium. The bowels should be kept fluid, and where the lesion has involved the bladder the catheter should be passed at least every six hours for five to six days. As is the rule for the puerperal state, the catheter must be passed by sight, and this is preceded by careful disinfection of the external genitals and the vestibule. If the sutures be aseptic they will not suppurate, and they should be left in place for fully two weeks. Should the primary operation fail, the woman should be advised to have the secondary operation performed without overmuch delay.

Rupture Of The Uterus. Rupture of the parturient uterus constitutes one of the most fatal as well as most alarming of the obstetric complications. There is scarcely an emergency which calls for more rapidity of judgment and of action; for, as will be noted, on prompt differential diagnosis and equally prompt treatment the life of the woman depends. The accident, fortunately, is an infrequent one, and will become all the more so as the benefits of strictly elective obstetric surgery become uniformly recognized.

The etiological factor cannot be always positively determined. In many instances rupture may be traced directly to the premature and injudicious administration of ergot; again, the causal factor is the attempt to drag a foetus through a pelvis where attention to the ordinary rules of pelvic mensuration will teach that delivery by one or another method is alone possible; further, a by no means infrequent factor has been protracted labor with consequent thinning of the lower uterine segment; and, finally, the operation of embryotomy through a greatlycontracted pelvis may be associated with rupture of the uterus. In certain instances none of these factors can be held responsible when, in default of a better reason, we must consider that the uterus has become weakened at a certain point, and has simply given way at the point of least resistance.

There are two varieties of rupture of the uterus, and on their differentiation depend both the prognosis and the treatment. These varieties are complete rupture and incomplete rupture.

The complete rupture is intra-peritoneal; the incomplete rupture is extraperitoneal. The clinical history will ordinarily enable the physician to differentiate the variety of rupture and the importance of accurate differentiation will shortly be apparent.

Incomplete rupture of the uterus may occur into either of the broad ligaments, or into the utero-vesical space, or into the *cul-de-sac* of Douglas. In any case the tear does not extend into the peritoneal cavity.

Complete rupture of the uterus necessarily invades the peritoneal cavity associated with, in general, the escape of the foetus in part or in whole into this cavity.

In incomplete rupture the shock is not as great and the loss of blood is limited by the capacity of the cavity into which it is effused.

In complete rupture with extrusion of the entire foetus into the peritoneal cavity the shock is great, and the haemorrhage which may take place is only limited by the amount of blood the patient has to lose. Where a portion only of the foetus is extruded, the amount of blood lost may be checked by the portion of the foetus which is not extruded acting as a tampon.

The signs which lead to diagnosis of rupture of the uterus are like those which are associated with haemorrhage. These signs will vary in intensity according as the haemorrhage is sudden and great or slow, even though gradually progressive. Shock, rapid pulse, pallor, sighing, eventually syncope,—such are the symptoms which should awaken the keen anxiety of the physician. The only positive way of making the differential diagnosis between complete and incomplete rupture is to insert the hand into the uterus, excepting, of course, in those instances where the foetus escapes into the peritoneal cavity, when, so to speak, the diagnosis is made for us.

If the rupture is incomplete, surgical treatment is not demanded, certainly at the outset. The proper course to pursue is one of expectancy. Where the rent extends from the angle of a lacerated cervix into the base of the broad ligament, the hemorrhage, in great part, comes from the circular artery, and this may be checked by carrying a suture around the artery and tying it. Where the rent involves the broad ligament or the anterior or the posterior *cul-de-mc,* the firm tamponade with sterilized gauze may check the hemorrhage and limit its extension. Often, however, the blood will continue to be effused until it has dissected the cellular tissue as far as its anatomical boundaries in the given region will allow. In other words, the condition becomes one of haematoma—ante-uterine, retro-uterine, or lateral—into the broad ligament. Later on, if the haematoma do not become absorbed, or if, through some faulty technique, suppuration set in, surgical interference may become necessary. Where the rupture is intra-peritoneal the prognosis, in any event, is most gloomy. If the foetus has escaped entirely or in greater part into the peritoneal cavity, the only possible operation is an abdominal section, not in the hope of saving the child, but in order to give the woman a single chance of life. There is no time in this emergency for special preparations. The physician must have the courage of his convictions; he must open the abdomen at once, extract the foetus, and treat the uterine rent by sewing it up after the manner pursued in the Caesarean section, or by removal of the entire uterus as is described under the Porro operation.

Where the rupture is complete, but the foetus has not escaped into the peritoneal cavity, there is scope for difference of opinion as to the proper treatment. The results from either of the methods which may be selected are the reverse of brilliant, although possibly of late years one of them has seemed to modify the prognosis for the better. At first thought, immediate emptying of the uterus and abdominal section would seem to be the desideratum. The fact is, however, that the woman, being in deep shock, abdominal section is simply superadding shock, and the wonder is when any recover. The alternate method is to rapidly extract the foetus and then to tampon the uterus with sterilized gauze; we thus compress the bleeding-point and perhaps check further loss of blood. Of late years a few cases treated after this fashion have recovered. If we are fortunate thus to check the haemorrhage, the peritoneum will take care of the blood which has escaped within it; and if the labor has been conducted aseptically and the gauze inserted is aseptic, then, if the woman do not die of shock, she will not die of sepsis. Resort to this method of tamponade is, however, only possible where the intestines have not protruded into the rent. If this has occurred, we cannot use the tamponade, because of the uncertainty as to whether or not the gut is strangulated at the uterine rent or through compression by the gauze. There can be no choice of procedure in case of intestinal prolapse; the physician's only recourse is abdominal section.

In case of incomplete rupture, where the tampon has been applied, the gauze should be left *in situ* for from thirty-six to sixty hours. Adjuvant treatment consists in raising the foot of the bed, bandaging the extremities, giving strychnia in large doses hypodermatically (grain every two hours, for its stimulating effect on the heart), and administering hot 2-per-cent. saline rectal injections.

A further and very rare form of uterine rupture is what is termed "annular rupture." This consists in separation of the cervix at the utero-vaginal junction, either in whole or in part. The treatment requisite is ligation of the circular arteries in the event of their being implicated in the rent.

We next pass to the consideration of the puerperal affections due to septic infection, which may require surgical aid. A point to be noted is that elective surgery is peculiarly applicable to these affections, since early treatment of this nature very frequently spares the woman results of the most untoward nature.

Endometritis And Metritis.

These affections are considered together because the one is the direct consequence of the other. On the prompt recognition of a septic endometritis depends the safety of the tubes, ovaries, peritoneum, and not infrequently the life of the woman. There has been, of late years, a radical change in the method of treatment of septic endometritis. The practice long in vogue, of repeatedly irrigating the uterus, has been found utterly inefficient as a means of guarding against infection of the Fallopian tubes, and thence of the peritoneal cavity. Whilst occasionally, when the local infection is slight and superficial, the repeated douche suffices to limit and to check extension of the process, we are never in a position to state definitely what cases will yield to this method, and, seeing that the aim is to check the septic process *in ovo,* so to speak, treatment of a more radical nature is favored by the majority of obstetricians, particularly since it may be definitely stated that such treatment, whilst most efficient for good, carries with it absolutely no risk to the patient when properly and aseptically performed.

The objections to which the douche is open are the following: No matter how often the douche is administered, all that it can accomplish is to wash the superficies of the endometrium. The germs at work on the surface are rendered inert, but those in the depths are not affected. To attempt to check a septic endometritis in this way is very much like trying to quench a fire by sprinkling water on it at intervals. Further, since the douches are always administered with the addition of some antiseptic, usually the bichloride of mercury, there is imminent risk of poisoning the woman, as numerous cases on record prove. Again, each additional manipulation to which the woman is subjected carries with it the risk of additional septic infection. Lastly, the repeated douche entails disturbance of a sick and nervous woman, and this is bad for the *morale* so necessary for convalescence from any affection, in particular where the disease is septic infection, when the aim of all therapeusis is to support the heart. For these cogent reasons the repeated douche has been given up by practically all accoucheurs. The following method, varied in only insignificant detail, has been substituted. On the appearance of foetor of the lochia, which, as a rule, is the precursor of developing septic endometritis, a vaginal douche is ordered, to certify to the fact that the foetor is not due to a vaginal source. If the foetor persist an intrauterine douche is administered, to exclude the presence of clots or loose fragments of decidua in the uterus. If the foetor then persist the time for action has come; for it must be borne in mind that, as yet, there may be no marked constitutional disturbance, such as chill or elevation of temperature, or even much elevation of the pulse-rate. Whenever possible the manipulations about to be described should be preceded by digital examination of the interior of the uterus, since not infrequently the symptoms awakening our suspicion are due to the retention of a piece of placenta which is beginning to necrose, or to portions of the membranes left behind. As a rule, it is not necessary to anaesthetize the woman; but if she is hyperaesthetic or peculiarly nervous, it is better to do so in order to lessen shock, as also in order to enable the procedure to be properly performed. The instruments necessary are a dull and a sharp curette with long handles, a vulsellum, a pair of intra-uterine packing-forceps, and a uterine irrigating-tube. A speculum is not strictly requisite, since the manipulations may be performed along the finger,—a practice necessary where the pelvic floor has been repaired. Thoroughness being requisite, however, the physician should never hesitate to sacrifice the restored pelvic floor, if necessary, in order to carefully explore the uterus.

Since it is desirable to avoid disturbing the woman as much as possible, we will describe the operation of curetting the puerperal uterus without the aid of the speculum. As a rule, also, we much prefer to use the sharp curette, since when the uterine mucosa is diseased it is absolutely essential to remove it in its entirety; for thus alone can we certainly eradicate the disease process and avoid a repetition of the operation. The risk we subject the woman to is slight compared with that she runs if the operation be not thorough. This risk is perforation of the uterus. If requisite care be used this risk is slight; still, it is desirable to have the friends of the woman distinctly understand that the procedure is not a minor one.

A fountain-syringe connected with a glass irrigating-tube or with a double-current intra-uterine catheter, and filled with a solution of 1 to 8000 bichloride of mercury, should be suspended within reach, and a pint bottle of peroxide of hydrogen should be opened. The hands of the operator, the instruments, and the external genitals of the woman should be thoroughly cleansed; the woman is brought to the edge of the couch and her legs are flexed on the abdomen. At the period of the puerperal state, when the manipulations about to be described are indicated, the cervical canal is open so that precedent dilatation will not be necessary. Again, whenever there is anything remaining in the puerperal uterus or whenever a septic process exists, the same state of the canal will be found. The index finger of the left hand is introduced into the vagina and placed at the external os. Along this finger the curette is guided into the uterus, absolutely no force being used, until the loop of the instrument reaches the fundus. If digital examination has revealed the presence of a portion of retained secundine or placenta undergoing degeneration, the instrument is guided to this and firm traction on the handle will remove it. Whilst the left hand is manipulating the handle of the curette, the right hand grasps the fundus of the uterus through the abdominal wall and not only controls it, but is ever conscious of the action of the curette. Herein lies a further value of the method of curetting without the speculum.

Where the entire endometrium is involved in the necrotic process, the curette, ever under the control of the external hand, should be made to traverse it, particular care being taken to explore the openings of the Fallopian tubes into the organ. When satisfied that the process is thoroughly eradicated, the curette is withdrawn, the irrigating-tube or the catheter is inserted and the uterine cavity is washed out, the antiseptic solution being at a temperature of about 115 F. When the fountain-syringe is empty, the peroxide of hydrogen is poured in and the uterine cavity is washed out with this. The catheter is now withdrawn; a strip of sterilized gauze, about two inches wide and eighteen inches long, is grasped by the packingforceps and carried into the uterus, the greater portion of the gauze being inserted. This insures free drainage externally.

As a rule, considerable depression follows these manipulations where anaesthesia has not been resorted to, and, therefore, it is generally desirable to use it. The gauze is left *in situ* from thirty-six to forty-eight hours, when, after renewed asepsis of the genitals and with aseptic hands the gauze is removed. The uterus is irrigated with hot 1 to 8000 bichloride, or with 2-percent, creolin, and a second strip of gauze is inserted, on this occasion not being packed in, but being placed more as a drain. If the curetting has been thorough it will rarely be necessary to repeat it; the local septic process is either at an end or it has extended to the parenchyma of the uterus, giving rise to a metritis, or to the tubes and ovaries, giving rise to a salpingitis or to an oophoritis. It is to avoid these untoward complications that it is essential to recognize a septic endometritis early, and to treat it radically after the manner just described.

Whilst the method of curetting through the speculum is not favored by us, since it is indorsed by many, we deem it essential to describe it. The additional instruments requisite are a speculum and a vulsellum forceps. If the operator prefer the Sims speculum, the woman is placed, of course, in the left lateral position, otherwise the Edebohl or the Simon speculum will answer for the dorsal position.

After due asepsis the cervix is exposed through the speculum, the vulsellum is made to grasp the anterior lip of the cervix, and the curette is inserted by sight instead of by touch. The manner of curetting is exactly similar to the process just described.

Frequently, after the curetting, the woman has a chill; but, as a rule, this has no significance, being entirely nervous in character. If, after the lapse of thirty-six hours, the temperature fall and the pulse approximate nearer the normal (and this fall of the pulse is the chief good omen), the chances are that the operation has been timely and that the woman has been spared extension to the parenchyma of the uterus or to the tubes and ovaries. If, on the other hand, the septic phenomena become intensified, then the physician must suspect extension, and his position must become an exceedingly alert one. A suppurative metritis or salpingo-odphoritis can be met in only one way, and this is through abdominal section. Even then the prognosis is most gloomy, since septic processes of this nature are ordinarily associated with deep systemic lymphatic absorption,—an affection against which our therapeutic resources, both medical and surgical, as yet avail but little. If, however, there should be reasonable doubt as to the systemic infection, the physician must not hesitate, but proceed to the one operation which offers the woman a single chance of life, and this is abdominal section with extirpation not alone of the purulent appendages, but also of the septic uterus. This seems a forlorn hope, and so it is; but the sole alternative in these aggravated types of sepsis is to allow the woman to die of septicaemia emanating from the uterus or the appendages, and this course of action is reprehensible, seeing that sometimes, although very rarely, even such desperate cases recover under the bold use of the knife.

Unfortunately, septic metritis, salpingitis, and oophoritis, when developing during the puerperium, are of such a virulent type and the associated general systemic infection is so profound that we can expect but one result, no matter what the therapeusis, and this result is death. The women die not so much because of the local lesions as because of the deep systemic infection. Still, since there are now and then recorded cases where aggressive surgery has resulted in ultimate recovery, in a given case the physician is bound to take into consideration the advisability of resorting to abdominal section. The steps of the operation are similar to those which are called for when total hysterectomy is performed for other causes. The object of the operation being to remove from the body the source of the systemic infection, ablation of the involved organs must be thorough; that is to say, the abdominal cavity having been opened, the entire uterus with the appendages must be removed in accordance with the steps which are laid down in modern treatises on gynaecology.

As a rule, there is associated with metritis and septic appendages the next subject we are called upon to consider:—

Puerperal Peritonitis. In considering this affection from a surgical standpoint, it is essential to note the change in practice which the last decade has witnessed, without, however, it must be confessed, any special change in secured results. It is a fact beyond dispute that, no matter what the form of treatment employed, the vast proportion of cases of puerperal peritonitis die. Large doses of opium, saline catharsis, abdominal section,—each of these approved methods has an exceedingly high mortality percentage. It must be remembered that puerperal peritonitis, whether local or general, is due to infection by one or two routes, aside from instances when peritonitis complicates the puerperal state, due to, we will say, rupture of an ovarian or tubal abscess or to a purulent appendicitis. The two modes of infection are either by direct extension from the uterine cavity or by lymphatic absorption. In the former instance the peritonitis is likely to be and to remain local; in the latter instance it is likely to become general. The systemic infection is by no means so exaggerated, as a rule, in local as in general purulent peritonitis. In general peritonitis the affection is secondary to general systemic infection. Not alone is the peritoneal cavity filled with multiple abscesses, but the lymphatics of the entire system are gorged with the infectious element and deposit it all over the body. The women die no matter what the form of treatment employed, not because of the peritonitis, but because of the deep general systemic infection. It is absolutely essential, therefore, to endeavor to differentiate local from general purulent peritonitis. Frequently this is possible; then, again, the symptomatology of the one suggests the other. The physical signs may be as aggravated, frequently more so, in instances of local as in cases of general peritonitis. And yet, no matter how extremely unfavorable the case may appear, sometimes speedy surgical action reveals a local instead of a general peritonitis, and sometimes the women recover.

So important is the factor of diagnosis that every means should be utilized toward reaching the desideratum,—a differential diagnosis between local and general peritonitis. Examination of the uterus with the finger to exclude septic focus there; palpation of the appendages, particularly by rectum, and, in case of doubt, with the assistance of deep surgical anaesthesia,— these and every other means should be used to clear the scene.

Notwithstanding all these differential diagnostic means, there are a certain proportion of cases where the physician will still remain in doubt as to whether he is dealing with a local or with a general peritonitis. Then, in remembrance of the fact that, if the affection be local although simulating general peritonitis, the woman's chance of life depends, in all probability, on his speedy action, gloomy as is the prognosis, it is his duty to resort to the single therapeutic measure which affords a gleam of hope. It must never be forgotten that surgery is full of surprises, and that our finite methods of diagnosis must often be supplemented and aided through resort to most desperate measures.

Local peritonitis presents itself under two forms,—as extraperitoneal and as incapsulated intra-peritoneal. The latter, however, is really extra-peritoneal in the sense that it is shut off from the general peritoneal cavity by adhesions, being originally intra-peritoneal. Etiologically the true extra-peritoneal exudate which may suppurate is not usually associated with tubal or ovarian infection, whilst the latter form is generally the sequela. This is the main reason why a true cellular abscess carries a less grave prognosis than the intra-and yet extra-peritoneal variety. The symptomatology of true pelvic abscess—that is to say, of abscess in the pelvic cellular tissue—may be as aggravated in type as the intra-peritoneal form; and yet the outcome of surgical treatment is much more favorable. Whenever the local and the general symptoms point to the existence of pus in the pelvic cellular tissue, the sooner it is evacuated the better. As a rule, the point of election for operating will be the vagina, since it is here that an abscess of this character usually points.

The operation is performed as follows: Thorough asepsis of the external genitals having been secured, under the guidance of the aseptic finger in the vagina an aspirator-needle is plunged into the softened exudate at a point close to the cervix, in order to avoid injuring the ureter. Along this aspirator-needle, as a guide, a narrow-bladed knife is passed and the opening into the cavity is enlarged. A steel-branched dilator is next inserted, and the opening is torn wider. The finger is then inserted into the cavity, and the different chambers which frequently go to make up the cavity are broken down. The cavity is then irrigated with bichloride or creolin solution, and next washed out with the full-volume peroxide of hydrogen. A T-shaped rubber drain-tube is then inserted, and through this the cavity is washed out daily until suppuration is at an end. If the cause of the symptoms has been the cellular abscess, in twenty-four to thirty-six hours the general condition of the woman will have altered materially for the better, and as soon as she has thrown off the general sepsis she will rapidly convalesce.

Such is the treatment and such the course of events in pure cellular abscess, which, we repeat, may present as aggravated symptoms as the intra-peritoneal variety, llarely these cellular abscesses do not point in the vagina, but above Poupart's ligament. Then the point of election for incision is at this site. The cavity is entered by an incision parallel to Poupart's ligament, is washed out after the same fashion, and, where possible, a counter-opening is made into the vagina, since thus we obtain better drainage, and, therefore, speedier convalescence.

It is the intra-extra-peritoneal variety of abscess which gives the most trouble, both from the diagnostic and the therapeutic stand-point. General purulent peritonitis, being an epiphenomenon of general septic infection, has as yet proven rebellious to every therapeutic measure. The woman dies not because she is suffering from peritonitis, but because she is deeply poisoned. The post-mortem findings explain this. Not only does the peritoneal cavity contain multiple abscesses, but the venous and lymphatic systems are similarly gorged.

AVhat then, it may reasonably be asked, is the use of surgical procedure-? Because, as we have already stated, the symptomatology of local peritonitis sometimes is suggestive of general peritonitis, and, therefore, abdominal section, even though the case appear of the most desperate type, may reveal a local peritonitis amenable to treatment. It must further be remembered that peritonitis, associated with purulent appendicitis, may complicate the puerperal state, and here prompt section may result in the saving of life. In this desperate disease one must have the courage of strong convictions, and operate, even though the battle seem lost before action. We are absolutely assured that nothing is to be gained from therapeutic nihilism, at any rate.

The abdominal cavity is opened in the usual way, and, if we are fortunate enough to find a local peritonitis instead of a general, the abscess-cavity is emptied, is washed out with peroxide of hydrogen (full strength), and is packed with sterilized gauze. If, however, the peritonitis is general and purulent, then the most we can do is to break up the multiple abscess-cavities as far as we can detect them, repeatedly flood the peritoneal cavity with hot sterilized water, and pack the lower part of the pelvis with gauze. If the woman recover, the result is fairly miraculous. If she die, the physician has the satisfaction of knowing that he has done his full duty by his patient and that the result was in no sense due to surgery.

Puerperal Mastitis.

In the light of our present knowledge, puerperal mastitis must be considered as due to infection. The germs or infectious material gain entrance through the lacteal ducts and cause the inflammatory process which may be aborted or which may suppurate.

In the latter event, we have the affection which is termed mammary abscess. Two varieties of mammary abscess are to be differentiated,—the glandular and the sub-glandular. The former is not specially uncommon; the latter is exceedingly so. The one is readily recognized; the other is not, running an insidious course and undermining the gland often before its presence is made sufficiently known to call for the recognized treatment.

Whilst much may be accomplished in the way of aborting suppuration through the use of the ice-bag, or, if the individual prefer, by hot applications, as soon as the physician is sure of the presence of pus, the earlier it is evacuated the better for the welfare of the breast. Glandular abscess ought to be recognized early; the reverse holds true in case of the sub-glandular variety. And yet this latter form is the one which always eventually does the most damage to the glandular tissue, and, besides, subjects the woman to the serious risk of perforation into the pleural cavity before there exists at times sufficient evidence of pus to justify incision. In these obscure cases, when, under the use of ice or heat, the cardinal symptoms of inflammation do not abate, exploration with the aspiratorneedle should be resorted to. Of course, this aspiration should be strictly aseptic, otherwise a non-suppurating exudation will be converted into a suppurating.

When the aspirator-needle reveals pus, or when there is evidence of pus without aspiration, the sooner the gland is incised the better. The line of incision should be radiating from the nipple outward, in order to avoid injuring more of the lacteal ducts than are already involved in the suppurative process. The affected breast should be scrubbed with soap and water, then with 1 to 8000 bichloride solution, and finally washed with sulphuric ether. With a clean knife an incision is made through the gland down to the abscess-cavity. When this has been opened, the finger is inserted in order to break up all the cavities into which the abscess is apt to be divided. After thorough irrigation with bichloride, the full-strength peroxide of hydrogen is poured in and the cavity is packed with sterilized gauze. A firm compression-binder is applied. At the end of twenty-four hours the dressing is removed, the cavity is again irrigated, a gauze drain is inserted, and a large sterilized sponge is placed over the breast.

A firm binder is applied over all. This method of compression secures close apposition of the abscess cavity-walls and prevents the further pocketing of pus. In the event of there being no evidence from the side of the pulse and the temperature of septic absorption, this second dressing need not be changed for a number of days, when the cavity may be found entirely closed.

In more complicated cases, where, for instance, a submammary abscess has not been recognized in its early stages, the pus may be found to have dissected the entire gland, and then all attempts to save the lacteal ducts are futile. As many counter-openings as are necessary, in order to secure efficient drainage, must be made, and every possible effort is requisite to prevent the pocketing of pus under the pectoral muscle and toward the pleural cavity.

As the principles of asepsis as applied not alone to the maternal breast, but also to the infant's mouth before it is applied to the breast, are understood by nurses and exacted by physicians, mammary abscess will become one of the rarest complications of the puerperal state. In large maternity hospitals, where the strictest care is required, the fact is that mammary abscess is now rarely met with, and, when it is, the nurse has been at fault, unless the mother has handled her breast with unclean hands.

CHAPTER IX. ECTOPIC GESTATION.

The subject of ectopic gestation is of prime interest to the general practitioner, for the reason that on his ability to recognize the condition *early* depends usually the life of his patient. Seeing that the majority of obstetric work falls within the province of the general practitioner, it seems appropriate that ectopic gestation should be considered from its therapeutic side in a work dealing with obstetric surgery.

We shall not enter into a discussion of the value of electricity in the treatment of ectopic gestation. Sufficient the statement that it seems proven that in its earlier stages the development of the ovum may be checked through the administration of galvanism or faradism. Our aim will be fulfilled when we have tersely noted the diagnostic points and have laid stress on the surgical treatment of ectopic gestation.

We shall consider this subject from the now generally accepted view that primarily all ectopic gestations are tubal. About the tenth week rupture of the tube occurs in one of two directions: (1) into the general peritoneal cavity; (2) into the broad ligament. In the latter event the gestation may or may not continue to term.

The surgery of ectopic gestation, therefore, envisages the subject from a number of stand-points: 1. Before tubal rupture. 2. After rupture (a) into the peritoneal cavity; *(b)* into the broad ligament. 3. During development to term. 4. At term and after term.

Essential to any treatment is accurate diagnosis. Before tubal rupture this will rarely be possible beyond strong hypothesis. At the time of rupture the symptomatology will ordinarily establish the diagnosis. During development to term and at term the diagnosis is often in doubt, not as to whether 13 (193) pregnancy exists, but as to whether it be uterine or extrauterine. After term, if the precedent history be clear, the diagnosis is established; but often it may be made only on abdominal section.

Before rupture—that is to say, before the tenth to twelfth week of gestation—the diagnosis may be reasonably predicated on the following history: A period of amenorrhoea, associated especially with the reflex disturbances of pregnancy, followed by irregular haemorrhages. Ordinarily there is a history suggestive of precedent disease of the uterus and appendages, and, as a rule, the woman has never conceived before or there has been a period of protracted sterility. On local examination (vaginal and rectal) the uterus is found enlarged, and one or the other tube as well (either *in situ* or posterior to the uterus). The woman, furthermore, often complains of sharp attacks of abdominal pain, which are the associates of the distension of the tube, or are due to peritoneal irritation from tearing of the peritoneal covering of the tube. This *ensemble* of symptoms should at once awaken the suspicion of the existence of tubal gestation. It is at this period that galvanism may be resorted to with safety, since it may do good and can only do harm in that its use postpones resort to surgery, if it do not render this unnecessary.

The symptoms of rupture vary according as the accident occurs into the peritoneal cavity or into the broad ligament. Accurate differentiation is essential, since there is but one possible line of action in the former event, and this is abdominal section as soon as feasible. The main symptom is collapse of varying degree, with the formation of a tumor in case of rupture into the broad ligament. Where the rupture is intraperitoneal, the symptoms suggestive of haemorrhage (fainting, sighing, rapid pulse, increasing pallor) are usually more grave than where the rupture is extra-peritoneal. The reverse may hold, however, since the intra-peritoneal bleeding may be gradual and the extra-peritoneal profuse. The precedent history, however, and the immediate symptoms should certify to the diagnosis almost always so as to lead to the adoption of the proper therapeusis, which is immediate abdominal section in case of intra-peritoneal haemorrhage, and expectancy in case of broad-ligament haemorrhage.

The symptomatology of ectopic gestation after primary extra-peritoneal rupture may be self-suggestive as regards diagnosis, and again may be very obscure. So long as the foetus is alive, the hearing of the heart-sounds and the perception of movements will certify as to pregnancy; but, usually, short of exploration of the uterus, normal gestation cannot be excluded. After l'eetal death, whilst the precedent history will suggest the likelihood of ectopic gestation, abdominal section alone, in the vast majority of cases, will clear the diagnosis.

The following conditions may simulate intra-peritoneal rupture of ectopic gestation: Abortion, dysmenorrhoea, rupture of some abdominal organ with escape of its contents into the peritoneal cavity, and pelvic peritonitis.

The following conditions may be mistaken for extra-peritoneal rupture of ectopic gestation: Intra-peritoneal rupture of the same condition, hematoma of the broad ligament from other causes, exudate in the cellular tissue of the ligament, and cyst of the broad ligament or abscess within it.

In both series of instances, attention to the history and careful physical examination, if need be under an anaesthetic, will often clear the diagnosis. Peritonitis may be excluded by the elevation of temperature, which exists, usually, from the outset. Exploration of the uterus, together with careful bimanual, *rectal* and *vaginal*, will exclude abortion, aside from the fact that shock rarely exists in the latter condition, except the woman be hyperaesthetic and hysterical, when it is never deep and progressive, but transient. In case of rupture of some viscus, such as the appendix vermiformis, with escape of its contents, where the depression is extreme, the therapeutic indication is the same as for rupture of a tubal pregnancy into the peritoneal cavity. The formation or the presence of a tumor in one or the other broad ligament, no matter what the condition, will lack the urgency calling for immediate surgery. Finally, there are instances where combined uterine and extrauterine gestation exist, and here, no matter how refined our diagnostic aids, the question can alone be settled by exploration of the uterus, and, in the event of supposed intra-peritoneal rupture, by abdominal section.

The diagnosis of ectopic gestation having been made with sufficient exactitude to swerve the judgment of two or more physicians in its favor, the woman must be regarded as subject to a greater or a less imminent risk, according to the period of gestation. The ovum is a parasite of ill omen to its mother, and its destruction or removal is called for when, by so doing, the immediate or the ultimate safety of the woman so requires.

Prior to tubal rupture, when the diagnosis is always uncertain, arrest of the growth of the ovum by means of galvanism or of faradism is justifiable. Absorption of so small a mass as the ovum is prior to the eighth or tenth week is perfectly possible, and, if this absorption should not occur, the woman at best is carrying a diseased tube, which at any time when it seems desirable may be removed by abdominal section. Where, however, the physician is a skilled operator, the immediate and future welfare of the woman is best secured through resort to abdominal section. The steps of the operation are the following: The abdomen and the pubes having been shaved and the integument having been cleansed by thorough scrubbing with soap and water, followed by 1 to 1000 bichloride solution, the woman is anaesthetized. The bladder is emptied. The instruments (scalpel, artery-forceps, ligature-carrier, Peaslee-Hagedorn needle) should be thoroughly sterilized, and the hands of the operator and of his assistants should be scrupulously cleansed. It must be remembered that septic infection is the sole risk the woman runs in the hands of an operator familiar with the technique.

The operation is likely to prove of shorter duration if the woman be placed in the Trendelenburg position. This position may be improvised by tying an ordinary kitchen-chair to the table so as to form the inclined plane. (See next page.)

In addition to the instruments, the operator should have prepared at least four large, flat, gauze pads and one dozen small gauze sponges. A quart-bottle full of 1-per-cent. hot (120 F.) sterilized salt-solution should be ready to irrigate the peritoneal cavity, in the event of threatened collapse from unavoidable haemorrhage. The peritoneum rapidly absorbs the salt-solution, and it forms our readiest restorative.

The usual incision is made down to the peritoneum, about three inches in length, extending upward from above the pubes. Any haemorrhage is checked by torsion of the small vessels.

Before opening the peritoneum the operator should emphasize his injunction that absolutely no antiseptics are to be used in the further progress of the operation.

The peritoneal cavity having been entered, one or more of the large gauze pads, wrung dry from the sterilized water, are inserted to keep the intestines from the abdominal opening. With one or two fingers the operator liberates the tube and ovary (if adherent) and brings them out of the abdominal incision. The ovarian artery being very vascular, it is desirable, when feasible, to isolate it and tie it separately with medium-sized sterilized silk. The pedicle is transfixed by the ligature-carrier; a stout, sterilized, Chinese-silk ligature is brought through, the ends are crossed and firmly tied, after the usual manner. The appendages are then removed.

The tube and ovary of the opposite side are next examined, and, if diseased, are similarly tied off.

The pads are now removed from the abdominal cavity. If the operation has not been associated with haemorrhage, it is not necessary to mop out or to irrigate the field of operation. In case the pulse is flagging, however, irrigation with the salt solution should be resorted to.

The abdominal incision is closed by deep silk-worm-gut

Fig. 84.—Emergency Trendelenburg Posture. (The inclined plane is formed by an ordinary chair being tied on a kitchen-table.)

sutures transfixing all the tissues and including carefully the fascia of the recti.

In the event of the woman not being seen until tubal rupture has occurred, the surgical treatment must be immediate if the haemorrhage be intra-peritoneal. The steps of the operation are similar to those just stated, except that, on opening the peritoneal cavity, no time should be lost in grasping the ruptured tube and tying it off, for this is the source of the haemorrhage. The peritoneal cavity should then be irrigated with hot, sterile salt-solution to act as a restorative and to wash out the major portion of the blood and clots. What must perforce be left behind the peritoneum will take care of, unless it be septic. Where this possibility is feared, drainage by gauze through Douglas's *cul-de-sac* is preferable to attempts at drainage through the abdominal incision.

When the diagnosis of rupture into

the broad ligament (extra-peritoneal rupture) has been reached the therapeusis should be strictly expectant; operative treatment is rarely called for. If the woman be kept in the recumbent position until the haematoma becomes smaller, but little other treatment will be necessary, beyond the self-suggestive means for meeting the greater or less acute anaemia from which the woman is suffering: such as frequent hot water (115 F.), saline (1 per cent.), rectal irrigation, strychnine hypodermatically (‚V grain every three to four hours), etc. Rarely the blood-clot breaks down into pus from septic infection. An opening should then be made into the sac from the vagina. The pus must be thoroughly evacuated, the sac washed out with the full-strength solution of peroxide of hydrogen, and drainage resorted to.

In a small proportion of cases the ovum survives the extraperitoneal rupture and continues to grow. The woman from now until term is in constant danger from the possibility of secondary rupture into the peritoneal cavity. Every day the increasing size of the child and of the placenta adds to the danger of this accident. The life of the woman alone is to be taken into consideration. The chances that development will continue and the child reach full term are small, and even if it should, and be safely removed, it rarely survives the first few weeks, and is rarely, also, perfectly formed.

Inasmuch as the continuous growth of the child constantly increases the danger which the woman must encounter, it is the duty of the physician to destroy it as soon as it has been determined that development is taking place. If development has continued beyond the fourth month, the death of the child will not increase the woman's safety. The sac may have formed adhesions with loops of intestine, and through this source sepsis may have entered the system. In such cases it is necessary to carefully watch the woman, and, as soon as any symptoms of sepsis are apparent, abdominal section is to be performed. These symptoms are chills, remittent temperature, rapid pulse. The sac is to be opened, the decomposed foetus is to be removed, and the opening of the sac is to be stitched to the abdominal wall. Usually the placenta will have become freed from its attachments and may be removed at the same time. Should it be adherent, however, it is preferable to allow it to come away in fragments. Free drainage should be maintained. Usually this operation will be practically extra-peritoneal.

If the child has reached full term and is alive, a very interesting complication calls for decision. The little notoriety which one gains from performing a brilliant operation should not influence the conscientious physician for a moment. Neither must sentimental notions carry the least weight in reaching a conclusion. The question to be decided is the following: "Should I operate and possibly save the life of the child, which at best will stand but few chances of surviving, and by so doing greatly add to the dangers of the already-unfortunate mother; or should I delay the operation and thereby permit the child to die and the placenta to lose very much of its vascularity, if, indeed, not all of it, and by this delay very much enhance the chance of recovery of the woman V To those who will look at this question purely from the stand-point of the woman, and who will consider, as they ought, the ectopic foetus as simply a parasite, the choice will unquestionably be in favor of delay. No one will deny the legitimacy or the imperative necessity of resorting to foeticide in the non-controllable vomiting of pregnancy, with the end in view of saving the woman. The belief of Tait, that those who advocate the killing of the child in developing extra-uterine pregnancy are simply "abortion-mongers," is illogical, and must be looked upon as one of those statements which are made in haste and are not retracted owing, possibly, to false pride.

After the child is dead and the placental circulation has ceased, operation carries far less danger to the woman. It is contended by some that no operation should be performed until symptoms supervene, but nature's tedious methods of relief and the many obvious dangers to which the woman must be exposed do not seem to justify non-interference. The abdomen should be opened as soon as the placental circulation has ceased (and this is certified to by the absence of placental murmur), the foetus is removed, and the sac is stitched to the abdominal wound. If the placenta is detached and lying free it should be removed, and the sac is drained and allowed to close from the bottom. If the placenta is adherent, no attempt should be made to free it, for it will come away gradually through the abdominal opening. Convalescence is hastened if a vaginal opening can be made at the same time and through-and-through drainage thus established.

Under the modern method of treatment we have outlined, ectopic gestation has been practically robbed of its terrors, and the almost absolute mortality rate of the past has been converted into the almost certain recovery rate of the present. Once again is the value of election in obstetric surgery certified.

INDEX.

Abortifacients, uselessness of, 58
Abortion, artificial, 34
in absolute pelvic contraction, 37
in case of haemorrhage, 39
in case of tumors, 38
in chorea, 36
in displacements of the uterus, 39
operation for the induction of, 41, 46
in pernicious anaemia, 36
in pernicious vomiting of pregnancy, 35
in pulmonary and cardiac disease, 34
in renal disease, 36
Abscess, mammary, 190
pelvic, 188
operation for, 188
Accouchement force-, 67
Accoucheur, asepsis of, 2
Anaemia, pernicious, artificial abortion in, 36
Anatomy of pelvis, 9
of symphysis pubis, 121
Antisepsis, 1
definition of, 2
Arm, prolapse of, method of rectifying,

107
   Arms, methods of delivery of, 111
Asepsis, 1
definition of, 2
of accoucheur and attendants, 2
of genital tract, 5
of hands and arms, 4
of instruments, 6
of ligatures and sutures, 7
of lying-in woman, 5
Axis-traction forceps, 73, 74
to the breech, 87
   Basiotribe, Tarnier's, 154
Beaudelocque, diameter of, 12
Bipolar version, 101
method of performing, 103
   Bladder, danger of injury to, in symphysiotomy, 123
   Braxton-Hicks method of version, 101
   Csesarean section, 133
abdominal suture after, 140
absolute indication, 132
dilatation of cervix after, 137
election in, 133
indications, 133
instruments for, 134
preparations for, 135
prognosis of, 144
relative indication, 132
statistical data, 145
suture of uterus after, 138
Catheter, Fritsch-Bozeman, 42
Cephalotribe, application of, 155
disadvantages of, 154
Lusk's, 154
Cephalotripsy, operation of, 153
Cervix, dilatation of, after Cajsarenn section, 137
lacerated, immediate repair of, 163
after-treatment, 167
contra-indications, 164
instruments necessary, 164
steps of operation, 165
suture material for, 164
manual dilatation of, 89, 102
multiple incision of, 89, 105
Chin, arrested at symphysis, extraction of, 116
Chorea, artificial abortion in, 36
Conjugate, diagonal, 13
true *(conjugata vera),* 14
Cranioclast, Braun's, 149
extraction by, 150
Craniotomy of the after-coming head,

152
of the before-coming head, 150
operation of, 148
Crotchet, 157
Curette, uterine, 41
   Decapitation, 157
delivery of head after, 159
method of performance, 158
   Decollator, Braun's, 158
   Diameters of fetal head, 16
of pelvis, external, 11
internal measurements of, 15
pelvic, increase in, by symphysiotomy, 122
transverse and oblique, 15
   Dilator, steel-branched. 41
Dilators, hydrostatic, 66
Dystocia, obstetric, 9
   Eclampsia, induction of labor in case of, 54
podalic version in, 97
Election, value of, in Csesarean section, 133
value of, in symphysiotomy, 121
Electricity as a means of inducing labor, 58
Elytrotomy, laparo-, 144
Embryotomy, 146
prognosis of, 161
Endometritis, curetting in, 182
gauze tampon in, 184
objections to douche in, 181
operation for, 183
post-operative treatment of, 185
puerperal, 181
Episiotomy, 83
Evisceration, 155
indications for and dangers of, 156
   Face presentations, low forceps in, 81
Fistulas, 174
after-treatment of, 176
operation for repair of, 176
Fcrtal head, diameters of, 16
   Foetus, determination of engagement of, 51
dimensions of, at term, 16
intra-uterine measurement of, 50
length of, 50
manual internal rotation of, 117
in case of occiput posterior, 118
Forceps, 72
anaesthesia for extraction by the, 77
application of low, 81
of medium, 88
   Forceps, compression by the, 75

contra-indications to the use of, 76
direction of traction in low, 83
Elliott's, 72
forces of the, 74
high, 91
Hunter's, 73
in breech presentations, 77
indications for the, 76
intra-uterine dressing, 45
introduction of left blade of, 79
introduction of right blade of, 80
Jewett's axis-traction, 74
leverage of the, 75
locking of, 80
low, in face presentations, 86
in occipito-posterior, 84, 85
Lusk-Tarnier, 73
medium, dangers of, 89
ovum, 42
position for the application of, 78
prognosis of, 92
Reynolds's traction rods for, 75
rotation by the, 75
to after-coming head, 116
to breech, 87
Funis, prolapse of, version in, 97
   Galbiati knife, objections to, 129
Gestation, ectopic, 193
broad ligament, rupture of, 195
treatment of, 196
development of, to term, 199
treatment, 200
diagnosis of, 193
at time of rupture, 194
before rupture, 194
intra-peritoneal rupture, 194
primary, 195
operation for primary rupture, 197
terminations of, 193
treatment after foetal death, 201
treatment of broad-ligament rupture, 199
   Glycerin, injections of, for inducing labor, 60
   Haemorrhage, artificial abortion in case of, 39
as a complication of symphysiotomy, 129
   Haemorrhage, induction of labor in case of, 53
Hands, asepsis of, 4
Head, after-coming, forceps to, 116
arrested at brim, extraction in case of, 115
delivery of, after decapitation, 159

foetal, arrested at symphysis 116
compressibility of, 51
on perineum, method of delivery of, 83
    Heart disease, artificial abortion in, 34
    Hook, blunt, 157
Hunter's low forceps, 73
Hysterectomy, laparo-, 141
after-treatment, 144
indications, 142
technique, 142
    Incision, multiple, of cervix, 89, 105
Incubator, 69
Instruments, asepsis of, 6
    Jewett's axis-traction forceps, 74
Justo-major pelvis, 18
Justo-minor pelvis, 19
    Kidney disease, artificial abortion in, 36
    Knife, Galbiati, 124
Krause's method for inducing labor, 61
    Kyphosis, 24
    Labor, premature, induction of, 47
in case of eclampsia, 54
in case of deformed pelves, 48
in case of haemorrhage, 53
method for, 58
prognosis of, 68
    Laparo-elytrotomy *(vide* Elytrotomy)
    Laparo-hysterectomy *(vide* Hysterectomy)
    Ligament, subpubic, necessity of cutting, in symphysiotomy, 126
    Ligatures, asepsis of, 7
Lusk-Tarnier forceps, 73
    Mastitis, glandular, 191
puerperal, 190
subglandular, 192
Membranes, puncture of, for inducing labor, 58
Mento-posterior position, symphysiotomy in, 127
Metritis, abdominal section in case of, 185
extension of sepsis causing, 184
puerperal, 181
    Nurse, asepsis of, 2
    Occipito-posterior position, forceps in, 84
manual rotation in, 118
symphysiotomy in, 127
    Oophoritis, septic, 186
    Osteomalacia, 28

Pelves, abnormal, 17
contracted, symphysiotomy in, 122
deformed, by tumors, 31
induction of labor in, 48
Pelvic version, elective, 96
Pelvimeters, 11
Pelvimetry, 11
digital, 13
Pelvis, anatomy of, 9
circumference of, 16
contraction of, artificial abortion in, 37
diameters of, increase in, by symphysiotomy, 122
external diameters of, 11
flat, rachitic, 23
flattened, 20
funnel-shaped, 28
internal diameters of, 13
justo-major, 18
justo-minor, 19
kyphotic, 24
Naegele, 30
oblique-ovate, 30
osteomalacic, 28
rachitic, 21
rachitic-scoliotic, 26
scoliotic, 25
spondylolisthetic, 27
transversely contracted, 24
    Perforator, Blot's, 148
scissors, 149
Perineorrhaphy, after-treatment, 173
contra-indications, 168
for complete rupture, 172
for partial rupture, 170
    Hoar's method of, 170
immediate, 107
instruments requisite for, 169
method of performing, 169
suture mntcrinl for, 171
Perineum, central laceration of, 173
laceration of, determination of, 168
varieties of laceration of, 168
Peritoneum, methods of infection of, 187
    Peritonitis, differentiation of local from general, 187
intra-peritonenl, encapsulated, 189
operation for, 190
local, 188
operation for, 188
puerperal, 186
Placenta previa, 53
bipolar version in, 102
Porro operation *(vide* Hysterectomy)

    Pregnancy, extra-uterine *(vide* Gestation, ectopic)
pernicious vomiting of, 35
Puerperium, surgery of, 163
Pulmonary disease, artificial abortion in, 34
    Quinine to promote contractions, 90
Rachitis, 21
    Reynolds's traction rods, 75
    Roberts's pelvis, 24
    Rotation, manual, of foetus, 117
    Salpingitis, septic, 186
Scoliosis, 25
    Specula, Simon's, 175
    Speculum, Edebohl's, 43
    Spondylolisthesis, 27
    Spondylotomy, 157
    Sponges, dangers of using, 7
    Suture, uterine, 138
Sutures, asepsis of, 7
    Symphysiotomy, 120
after-treatment of, 128
amount of gain in diameters by, 122
anatomical considerations, 121
complications of, 128
delivery after, 126
factors controlling, 123
Galbiati knife for, 124
indications, 122
instruments essential for, 124
prognosis of, 130
repair of wound after, 127
statistical data, 130
structures involved in, 122
technique of, 124
subcutaneous method, 125
ultimate results from, 129
Symphysis pubis, effect of operation at, 129
mobility at, 128
    Tenaculum, cervical, 43
Trephine, Braun's 148
.Martin's, 149
Tumors, deforming the pelvis, 31
pelvic, artificial abortion in, 37
Twins, locked, 161
    Urethra, danger of injury to, in symphysiotomy, 123
Uterus, displacements, artificial abortion in, 39
management of, after Cesarean section, 136
rupture of, 177
abdominal section in, 179

annular, 181
prognosis of, 179
suture of, after Ca;sarean section, 138
tamponade in, 180
treatment of, 178
varieties of, 177
   Vagina, asepsis of, 5
hand in, for purpose of examination, 99
tamponing, for inducing labor, 59
Vaselin, dangers in using, 6
   Version, 93
bipolar, in case of placenta praevia, 10'2
   Braxton-Hicks method, 101
by external manipulations, 101
cephalic, 94
combined method of, 101
internal, 105
extraction after, 110
extraction of head, 112
insertion of hand in, 106
rotation of foetus by, 94
seizure of foot in, 107
ersion, liberation of arm after, 111
nomenclature of, 94
pelvic, 94
objections to, 100
performance of cephalic, 95
podalic, 96
contra-indications of, 97
indications for, 97
preparations for, 99
prognosis of, 119
varieties of, 94

   Catalogue of the Publications of THE F. A. DAVIS CO., JVIedleal Publishers and Booksellers,
1914 and 1916 CHERRY STREET, Philadelphia, Pa.
   Branch Offices: NEW YORK CITY—117 W. Forty-Second Street. CHICAGO 9 Lakeside Building, 214-220 8. Clark Street.
F. J. REBMAN, 11 Adam St., Strand, W.C. , London, Eng.
Order From Nearest Office.
   For Sale By All Booksellers.
   Prices of books, as given in our catalogue or circulars, include full prepa3'ment of postage, freight, or express charges. Customers in Canada and Mexico must pay the cost of duty, in addition, at point of destination.

   We do not hold ourselves responsible for books sent by mail; to insure safe arrival of books sent to distant parts, the package should be registered. Charges for registering (at purchaser's expense), 8 cents for every four pounds or less.
   N.B.—Remittances should be made by Express MoneyOrder, Post-Omco Money-Order, Registered Letter, or Draft on New York City, Philadelphia, Boston, or Chicago. Money sent in any other way must be entirely at risk of sender.
   The ATTENTION OF MEDICAL STUDENTS PARTICULARLY is
DIRECTED TO THE FOLLOWING STANDARD TEXT-AND
REFERENCE-BOOKS ANNOUNCED IN THIS CATALOOUE:
CATHELL—Book on the Physician Himself. Puge 2.
DAVIS—Diseases of Lungs, Heart, and Kidneys. Page 3. EDINOER—The Structure of the Central Nervous System. Page 3.
ElSENBERQ—Bacteriological Diagnosis. Page 3.
OOODELL— Lessons in Oymecology. Page 4. ORANDIN and JARHAN—Obstetric Surgery. Page 4.
International System of Electro-Therapeutics. Page 5.
IVINS— Diseases of the Nose and Throat. Page 5. LIEBIO and ROHE—Electricity In Hedlcine and Surgery. Page 0. riANTON—Syllabus of Lectures on Human Embryology. Page 6. PURDY—Practical Uranalysls and Urinary Diagnosis. Page 8. ROHE—Text-Book of Hygiene. Page 9. ROHE—Practical rianual of Skin Diseases. Page 9. SENN—Principles of Surgery. Page 9. SHOEriAKER—Hateria Itedlca and Therapeutics. Page 10.
SnlTH—Physiology of the Domestic Animals. Page 10.
STEWART—Obstetric Synopsis. Page 11. YOUNQ—Synopsis of Human Anatomy. Page 12. KRAFFT-EBINO—Psychopathla Sexualis. Page 13. RANNEY—Lectures on Nervous Diseases. Page 13. SAJOUS—Lectures on Diseases of the Nose and Throat. Page 13.
The above books can be examined and obtained at address given on Title-page of this Catalogue, and of booksellers generally.
   Catalogue of the Publications of THE F. A. DAVIS CO., ledieal Publishers and Booksellers, PHIUADHUPHIK, U. S. A.
   Publications distinguished by an asterisk () are issued in London, England, by f. J. Rebman, and in most cases have to be imported.
BALLIN—Personal Hygiene.
   By Mrs. Ada S. Ballin, Editor of "Baby; the Mothers' Magazine." Crown Octavo. About 250 pages. Cloth.
   Price, in United States and Canada, 60 cts., net; Great Britain,
3s..6d.; France, 4 fr.
BASHORE—Improved Clinical Chart.
   For the Separate Plotting of Temperature, Pulse, and Respiration. But one color of ink necessary. Designed for the Convenient, Accurate, and Permanent Daily Recording of Cases in Hospital and Private Practice. By Harvey B. Bashore, M.D. Fifty Charts, in Tablet Form. Size, 8 x 12 inches.
   Price, in United States and Canada, 50 cts., net; Great Britain, 3s. 6d.; France, 3 fr. 60.
BOENNING—Text-Book on Practical Anatomy.
   Including a Section on Surgical Anatomy. By Henry C. Boennino, M. D., Demonstrator of Anatomy in the Medico-Chirurgical College, etc. About 200 WoodEngravings. Royal Octavo. Nearly 500 pages. Extra Cloth. Also in Oil-Cloth, for use in the dissecting-room without soiling.
   Price, in United States and Canada, S2.50, net; Great Britain, 14s.; France, 16 fr. 20.
BOUCHARD—Auto-Intoxication.
   Being a series of lectures on Intestinal and Urinary Pathology. By Prof. Ch. Bouchard, Paris. Translated from the French, with an Original Appendix, by Thomas Oliver, M.A., M.D., Professor of Physiology, University of Durham, England. Over 300 pages. Crown Octavo. Extra Cloth.
   Price, in United States and Canada, SI.75, net; Great Britain, 10.;
France, 12 fr. 20.
BOWEN—Hand-Book of Materia Medi-

ca, Pharmacy, etc.

By Cuthbkrt Bowen, M.D., B.A. ISmo. 370 pages. Extra Cloth.

Price, in United States and Canada, S1. 40, net; Great Britain, 8. 6d.; France, 9 fr. 2S.

Medical Publications of The F. A. Davis Co., Philadelphia. BURET—Syphilis in Ancient and Prehistoric Times.

With a chapter on the Rational Treatment of Syphilis in the_ Nineteenth Century. By Dr. F. Buret, Paris, France. Translated from the French, with the author's permission, with notes, by A. H. Oumann-dumesnil, M.D., Bt. Louis, Mo. 230 pages. 12mo. Extra Cloth. This volume is one of a series of three. The other two, treating of Syphilis in the Middle Ages and in Modern Times, are now in active preparation.

Price, in United States and Canada, S1.25, net; Great Britain, 6s. 6d.; France, 7 fr. 76.

CAPP—The Daughter.

Her Health, Education, and Wedlock. Homely Suggestions to Mothers and Daughters. By William M. Capp, M.D., Philadelphia. 12mo. 150 pages. Attractively bound in Extra Cloth.

Price, in United States and Canada, S1.00, net; Great Britain, 6s.; France, 6 fr. 20. In Paper Covers (unabridged), 50 ets., net.

CATHELL—Book on the Physician Himself.

And Things that Concern his Reputation and Success. By D. W. Cathell, M.D., Baltimore, Md. Tenth Edition. Author's last revision. Royal Octavo. About 360 pages. Extra Cloth.

Price, in United States and Canada, S2.00, nct; Great Britain, 1fl. 6d.; France, 12 fr. 40.

CLEVENGER—Spinal Concussion.

Surgically Considered as a Cause of Spinal Injury, and Neurologically Restricted to a Certain Symptom Group, for which is Suggested the Designation "Erichsen's Disease," as one form of the Traumatic Neuroses. By S. V. Clevenoer, M.D., Consulting Physician, Reese and Alexian Hospitals; Late Pathologist, County Insane Asylum, Chicago, etc. Royal Octavo. Nearly 400 pages. With SO WoodEngravings.

Price, in United States and Canada, S2.50, net; Great Britain, 14s.; France, 15 fr.

COLT/IAN—The Chinese: Their Present and Future.

Medical, Political, and Social. By Robert Coltman, Jr., M.D., Surgeon in Charge of the Presbyterian Hospital and Dispensary at Teng Chow Fu, etc. Fifteen Fine Engravings on Extra Plate Paper, from photographs of persons, places, and objects characteristic of China. Royal Octavo. 212 pages. Extra Cloth, with Chinese Side-Stamp in gold.

Price, in United States and Canada, S1.75, net; Great Britain, 10s.; France, 12 fr. 20.

DAVIS—Diseases of the Lungs, Heart, and Kidneys.

By N. S. Davis, Jr., A.M., M.D., Professor of Principles and Practice of Medicine, Chicago Medical College, etc. 12mo. Over S00 pages. Extra Cloth.

Price, in United States and Canada, 1. 25, net; Great Britain, 6s. 6d.; France, 7 fr. 75.

Medical Publications of The F. A. Davis Co., Philadelphia. DAVIS—Consumption: How to Prevent it and How to Live with it.

Its Nature, Causes, Prevention, and the Mode of Life, Climate, Exercise, Food, and Clothing Necessary for its Cure. By N. 8. Davis, Jr., A.M., M.D. 12mo. 143 pages. Extra Cloth.

Price, in United States and Canada, 75 ots., net; Great Britain, 4s.; France, 4 *tr.*

DEMARQUAY—On Oxygen.

A Practical Investigation of the Clinical and Therapeutic Value of the Gases in Medical and Surgical Practice, with Especial Reference to the Value and Availability of Oxygen, Nitrogen, Hydrogen, and Nitrogen Monoxide. By J. N. DekarQUAY, Surgeon to the Municipal Hospital, Paris, and of the Council of State, etc. Translated, with notes, additions, and omissions, by Samuel S. Wallian, A.M., M.D., ex-President of the Medical Association of Northern New York, etc. Koyal Octavo. 316 pages. Illustrated with 21 Wood-Cuts.

Price, in United States and Canada, Cloth, 2.00, net; Half-Russia. S3.00, net. Great Britain, Cloth, 1is. 6d.; Half-Russia, 17s. 6d. France, Cloth, 12 fr. 40; Half-Russia, 18 tr. 60.

EDINOER—Structure of the Central Nervous System.

For Physicians and Students. By Dr. Ludwig Edinokr, Frankfort-on-theMain. Second Revised Edition. With 133 illustrations. Translated by Willis Hall Vittum, M.D., St. Paul, Minn. Edited by C. Eugene Riggs, A.M., M.D., Professor of Mental and Nervous Diseases, University of Minnesota, etc. Royal Octavo. About 250 pages. Extra Cloth.

Price, in United States and Canada, S1.75, net: Great Britain, 10s.; France, 12 fr. 20.

EISENBERQ—Bacteriological Diagnosis.

Tabular Aids for use in Practical Work. By James Eisenberg, Ph.D., M. D., Vienna. Translated and augmented, with the permission of the author, from the second German Edition, by Norval H. Pierce, M.D., Chicago, 111. Nearly 200 pages. Royal Octavo, bound in Cloth and in Oil-Cloth (for laboratory use). Price, in United States and Canada, S1.50, net; Great Britain, 8s. 6d.; France, O fr. 35.

FIREBAUQH—The Physician's Wife.

And the Things that Pertain to Her Life. By Ellen M. Firebaugb. Gracef ally written, full of genuine humor, and true to nature, this little volume is a treasure that will lighten and brighten many an hour of care and worry. Crown Octavo, 200 pages, with 44 Original Character Illustrations and a Frontispiece Portrait of the Author. Extra Cloth. Price, S1.25, net; Great Britain, 6s. 6d.

Special Limited Edition—First 500 copies beautifully printed in Photogravure Ink on Extra-Quality Enameled Paper, with wide margins, showing the illustrations with excellent effect. Beautifully and attractively bound in Fine Vellum Cloth and Leather. Price, S3.00, net. The Publishers reserve the right to increase this price without notioe.

GANT and ALLINQHAM—Diseases of Rectum and Anus.

By S. G. Gant, M.D., Professor of Rectal and Anal Surgery in the University Medical College, Kansas City; Lecturer on Rectal and Anal Diseases in the Scarritt Training School and Hospital for Nurse, etc.; and H. W. Allinoham, M.D. Surgeon to the Great Northern Hospital, and Junior Surgeon to St. Mark's Hospital for Rectal Diseases, London, etc. With numerous Illustrations, including several Full-page Colored Photo-engravings. Royal Octavo. In Preparation.

GOODELL—Lessons in Gynaecology.

By William Goodeli., A.M., M.D., etc.. Professor of Clinical Gynecology in the University of Pennsylvania. With 112 Illustrations. Third Edition, thoroughly revised and greatly enlarged. One volume. Large Octavo. 578 pages.

Price, in United States and Canada, Cloth, S5.00; Full Sheep, K6.00.

Discount, 20 per cent., making it, net, Cloth, S4.00; Sheep, S4.80.

Postage, 27 cents extra. Great Britain, Cloth, 22s. 6d.; Sheep, 28s. Franee, 30 fr. 80.

GRANDIN and JARHAN—Obstetric Surgery.

By Egbert H. GrAndin, M.D., Obstetric Surgeon to the New York Maternity Hospital; Gynaecologist to the French Hospital, etc.; and George W. Jarman, M.D., Obstetric Surgeon to the New York Maternity Hospital; Gynaecologist to the Cancer Hospital, etc. With about 85 Illustrations in the text and 15 Full-page Photographic Plates. Royal Octavo. About 250 pages. Extra Cloth.

Price, in United States and Canada. S2.50, net; Great Britain, 14s.; France, 15 fr.

OUERNSEY—Plain Talks on Avoided Subjects.

By Henry N. Guernsey, M.D., formerly Professor of Materia Medica and Institutes In the Hahnemann Medical College of Philadelphia, etc. Contents of the Book—I. Introductory. II. The Infant. III. Childhood. IV. Adolescence of the Male. V. Adolescence of the Female. VI. Marriage: The Husband. VII. The Wife. VIII. Husband and Wife. IX. To the Unfortunate. X. Origin of the Sex. 16mo. Bound in Extra Cloth.

Price, in the United States and Canada, S1.0O; Great Britain, 6s.; France, 6 fr. 20.

HARE—Epilepsy: Its Pathology and Treatment.

By Hobart Amory Hare, M.D., B.Sc, Professor of Materia Medica and Therapeutics in the Jefferson Medical College, Philadelphia, etc. 12mo. 228 pages. Extra Cloth.

Price, in United States and Canada, 91.25, net; Great Britain, fis. 6l.; France, 7 fr. 75.

HARE—Fever: Its Pathology and Treatment.

Containing Directions and the Latest Information Concerning the Use of the So-called Antipyretics in Fever and Pain. By Hobart Amory Hare, M.D., B. Sc. Blustrated with more than 25 new plates of tracings of various fever cases, showing the action of the antipyretics. The work also contains 85 carefully-prepared statis. tlcal tables of 249 cases, showing the untoward effects of the antipyretics. 12mo Extra Cloth.

Price, in United States and Canada, S1.25, net; Great Britain, 6s. 6d.; France, 7 fr. 75.

Medical Publications of The F. A. Davis Co., Philadelphia. HUIDEKOPER—Age of the Domestic Animals.

Being a Complete Treatise on the Dentition of the Horse, Ox, Sheep, Hog, anil Dog, and on the various other means of determining the age of these animals. By Rush Shipprn Huidekoper, M.D., Veterinarian (Alfort, France); Professor of Sanitary Medicine and Veterinary Jurisprudence, American Veterinary College, New York, etc. Royal Octavo. 225 pages. 200 Wood-Engravings. Extra Cloth.

Price, in United States and Canada, S1-75, net; Great Britain, 10a.; France 12 fr. 20.

International System of Electro-Therapeutics.

For Students, General Practitioners, and Specialists. Chief Editor, HORATIO R. Bigelow. M.D., Fellow of the American Electro-Therapeutic Association; Member of tho Philadelphia Obstetrical Society; Member of the Socie-te Francalse d'Electro-Therapie; Author of "Gynaecological Electro-Therapeutics," and "Familiar Talks on Electricity and Batteries," etc. Assisted by thirty-eight eminent specialists in Europe and America as associate editors. Thoroughly Illustrated with many tine Engravings. 1160 pages. Royal Octavo.

Price, in United States and Canada, Extra Cloth, S6.00, net; Sheep,

S7.00 net; Half-Russia, S7.50, net. In Great Britain, Cloth, 34s.

Sheep, 38s.; Half-Russia, 42s. In France, Cloth, 38 fr. 40; Sheep, 44 fr. 45; Half-Russia, 48 fr. 20.

IVINS—Diseases of the Nose and Throat.

A Text-Book for Students and Practitioners. By Horace F. Ivins, M.D., Lecturer on Laryngology and Otology, Hahnemann Medical College of Phila., etc. Royal Octavo. 507 pages. With 129 Illustrations, chiefly original, including 18 Colored Figures from Drawings and Photographs of Anatomical Dissections, etc. Price, in United States and Canada, Extra Cloth, S4.00, net; Sheep or Half-Russia, S5.00, net. Great Britain, Cloth. 22s. 6d.; Sheep or Half-Russia, 28s. Fiance, Cloth, 24 fr. 60; Sheep or Half-ItuBsla, 30 fr. 30.

JOAL—On Respiration in Singing.

For Specialists, Singers, Teachers, Public Speakers, etc. By Dr. Joal (Mont Dore). Translated and edited by R. Nokris Woi.fenden, M.D.Cantab., Editor of the Journal of Laryngology, etc. ; Vice-President of the British Laryngological Association, etc. In Active Preparation. Nearly Ready. Illustrated. Cloth. Crown Octavo. About 240 pages.

KEATING—Record-Book of Medical Examinations for LifeInsurance.

Designed by John M. Keating, M.D. This record-book Is small, bnt complete, and embraces all the principal points that are required by the different companics. It is made in two sizes, viz: No. 1, covering one hundred (100) examinations, and No. 2, covering two hundred (200) examinations. The size of the book is 7 %S% inches, and can be conveniently carried in the pocket.

Prices: No. 1, United States and

Canada, Cloth, 50 cents, net; Great Britain, 3s. M.; France, 3 fr. 60. No. 2, Full Leather, with Side-Flap, United States and Canada, S1.0O, net; Great Britain, 6b. 6d.; France, 6 fr. 20.

Medical Publications of The F. A. Davis Co., Philadelphia. KEATING and EDWARDS—Diseases of the Heart and Circulation in Infancy and Adolescence.

With an Appendix entitled "Clinical. Studies on the Pulse in Childhood." By John M. Keating, M.D., Philadelphia, and William A. Edwards, M.D.. Philadelphia. Illustrated by Photographs and Wood-Engravings. About 225 pages. 8vo. Hound in Cloth.

Price, In United States and Canada, S1.50, net; Great Britain, 8s. 6d.; France, 9 fr. 35.

KRAFFT-EBINQ—A Text-Book on Insanity.

For the Use of Students and Practitioners. By Dr. R. Von Krafft-ebing, Authorized translation of the Fifth German Edition by Ciiaki.es Gilbert Ciiadi-ioCK, M.D., Professor of Nervous and Mental Diseases in Marion-Sims College of Medicine, St. Louis, Mo., etc. Royal Octavo. About 800 pages. In Preparation. LIEBIG and ROHE—Electricity in Medicine and Surgery.

By G. A. Liebig, Jr., Ph.D., Assistant in Electricity, Johns Hopkins University, etc.; and Gkoroe II. Roue, M.D., Professor of Obstetrics and Hygiene, College of Physicians and Surgeons, Baltimore. Profusely Illustrated by WoodEngravings and Original Diagrams. Royal Octavo. 383 pages. Extra Cloth.

Price, in United States and Canada, S2.00, net; Great Britain, 1is. 6d.; France, 12 fr. 40.

flANTON—A Syllabus of Lectures on Human Embryology.

An Introduction to the Study of Obstetrics aud Gynaecology, with a Glossary of Embryological Terms. By W-altkk Porter Manto.n, M.D., Lecturer on Obstetrics in Detroit College of Medicine; Fellow of the Royal Microscopical Society, of the British Zoological Society, etc. Interleaved for taking notes, and thoroughly Illustrated by Outline Drawings and Photo-Engravings. 2mo. About 125 printed pages, besides the blank leaves for notes. Extra Cloth.

Price, in United States and Canada, S1.25, net; Great Britain, 6s. 6d.; France, *1 lt. 16.*

MASSEY—Electricity in the Diseases of Women.

With Special Reference to the Application of Strong Currents. By G. Button MASSEY, M.D., Late Electro-Therapeutist to the Philadelphia Orthopaedic Hospital and Infirmary for Nervous Diseases, etc. Second Edition. Revised and Enlarged. With New and Original Wood-Engravings. Extra Cloth. 240 pages. 12uio.

Price, in United States and Canada, SI.50, net; Great Britain, 8s. 6d.; France, 9 fr. 35.

iledical Bulletin Visiting List, or Physicians' Call Record.

Arranged upon an Original and Convenient Monthly and Weekly Plan for the Daily Recording of Professional Visits. Handsomely bound in fine strong Leather, with flap, including a Pocket for loose Memoranda, etc. Furnished with a Dixon lead-pencil of excellent quality and finish. Compact and convenient for carrying in the pocket. Size, 4 x 67,, inches. In three styles. *Send for deteripiive circular.*

No. 1. For 70 patients daily each month for one year, S1.25, net.
No. 2. For 105 patients daily each month for one year, S1.50, net.
No. 8. In which " The Blanks for Recording Visits in" are in six (6) removable sections, S1.75, net. Special Edition for Great Britain only, 4s. 6d.

Medical Publications of the F. A. Davis Co., Philadelphiu. nICHENFR—Hand-Book of Eclampsia.

Or, Notes and Cases of Puerperal Convulsions. By E. Michener, M.D.; J. H. Stubbs, M.D.; K. B. Ewing, M.D.; B. Thompson. M.D.; S. Stebbins, M.D. 16ino. Cloth. Price, 60 cts , net. Great Britain, 3s. 6d.

nONTQOMERY—Practical Gynaecology.
By E. E. Montgomery, A.M., M.D, Professor of Clinical Gynaecology in the Jefferson Meilical College, Philadelphia, etc., etc. In one Royal Octavo volume. Thoroughly Illustrated. In Preparation. MOORE—rieteorology.

By J. W. Moore, B. A., M.Ch., University of Dublin; Fellow and Registrar of tho Royal College of Physicians of Ireland, etc. Part L Physical Properties of the Atmosphere. Part II. A Complete History of the United States Weather Bureau from its Beginning to the Present Day, specially contributed by Prof. W. M. Harrington, Chief of the Weather Bureau in Washington, D. C., giving also a full list of all the stations under the immediate control of tho United States Government. Part III. Weather and Climate. Part IV. The Influence of Weather and Season on Disease. Profusely Illustrated throughout. One volume. Crown Octavo. Over 400 pages. Cloth.

Price, post-paid, in United States and Canada, S2.00, net; Great Britain, 8s.; France, 0 fr. 50.

MYGIND—Deaf-Mutism.

By Holder Mygind, M.D., of Copenhagen. The only authorized English Edition. Comprising Introduction, Etiology and Pathogenesis, Morbid Anatomy, Symptoms and Sequelae, Diagnosis, Prognosis, and Treatment. Crown Octavo. About 300 pages. Cloth.

Prico, post-paid, in United States and Canada, S2.00, net; Great Britain, 8s.; France, 9 fr. 50.

NISSEN—A Manual of Instruction for Giving Swedish
Hovement and Massage Treatment.

By Prof. Hartvig Nissen, lata Instructor in Physical Culture and Gymnastics at the Johns Hopkins University, Baltimore, Md., etc. With 29 Original Wood-Engravings. 12mo. 128 pages. Cloth.

Price, in United States and Canada, si.oo, net; Great Britain, 6s.; France, 6 fr.!J0.

Physicians' All-Requisite Time-and Labor-Saving
Account-Book.

Being a I-cdgcr and Account-Book for Physicians' Use, meeting all the Requirements of the I.aw and Courts. Designed by William A. Keibert, M.D., of Easton, Pa. There is no exaggeration in stating that this Account-Book and Ledger reduces the labor of keeping physicians' accounts more than one-half, and at the same time secures the greatest degree of accuracy.

Prices: No. 1, 300 pages for 900 Accounts per Year, size 10 x 12, bound in ¾-Russia, Raised Back-Bands, Cloth Sides, in United States and Canada, S6.00, net; Great Britain, 28s.; France, 30 fr. 30.

No. 2, 600 pages for 1800 Accounts per Year, size 10 x 12, bound in ¾-Russia. Raised Back-Bands, Cloth Sides, in United States and Canada, S8.00; Great Britain, 42s.; France, 49 fr. 40.

Send for descriptive circular showing the plan of the book.

Medical Publications of The F. A. Davis Co., Philadelphia.

Physicians' Interpreter.

In Four Languages, English, French, German, and Italian. Specially arranged for diagnosis by M. von V. The plan of the book is a systematic arrangement of questions upon the various branches of Practical Medicine, and each question is so worded that the only answer required of the patient is merely Yes 0i No. Bound In full Russia Leather, for carrying in the pocket. Size, 5x2⅞ inches. 206 pages. Price, in United States and Canada, «1.00. net; Great Britain, 6«.; France, 6 fr. 20.

PURDY—Diabetes.

Its Cause, Symptoms, and Treatment. By Chas. W. Purdy, M.D., Honorary Fellow of the Royal College of Physicians and Surgeons of Kingston; Author of "Bright's Disease and Allied Affections of the Kidneys"; Member of the Association of American Physicians; Mcmher of the American Medical Association, etc., etc. With Clinical Illustrations. 12mo. 184 pages. Extra Cloth.

Price, in United States and Canada, S1.25, net; Great Britain, 6s. 6d.; France, 7 fr. 75.

PURDY—Practical Uranalysis and Urinary Diagnosis.

A Manual for the Use of Physicians and Students. By C1iA8. W. PCRDY, M. D., Author of "Diabetes: its Cause, Symptoms, and Treatment"; Member of the Association of American Physicians, etc., etc. With numerous Illustrations, including several Colored Plates. Crown Octavo. About 350 pages. Extra Cloth. Price, in United States and Canada, S2.50, net. Great Britain, 14s.; France, 16fr.20.

REflONDINO—History of Circumcision. From the Earliest Times to the Present. Moral and Physical Reasons for its Performance; with a History of Eunuchism, Hermaphrodism, etc., and of the Different Operations Practiced upon the Prepuce. By P. C. Remondino, M.D., Member of the American Medical Association, of the American Public Health Association; Vice-President of California State Medical Society, etc 12mo. 348 pages. Extra Cloth. Illustrated with two fine full-page Wood-Engravings, showing the two principal modes of Circumcision in ancient times.

Price, in United States and Canada, S1.25, net; Great Britain, 6s. 6d.; France, 7 fr. 75. A Popular Edition (unabridgod), bound in Paper Covers, is also issued. Price, 60 cents, net; Great Britain, 3s.; France, 3 fr. 60.

REflONDINO—The flediterranean Shores of America.

Southern California: its Climatic, Physical, and Meteorological Conditions. By P. C. Remondino, M.D. Royal Octavo. 175 pages. With 45 appropriate Illustrations and 2 finely-executed Maps of the region, showing altitudes, ocean currents, etc. Bound in Extra Cloth.

Price, in United States and Canada, S1.25, net; Great Britain, 6s. 6d.; France, 7 fr. 75. Cheaper edition (unabridged), bound in Paper, in United States and Canada, 75 cts., net; Great Britain, 4s.; France, 5 Tr.

ROBINSON and CRIBB—The Law and Chemistry Relating to Food.

A Manual for the Use of persons practically interested in the Administration of the Law relating to the Adulteration and Unsoundness of Food and Di ugs. By H. Mansfield Robinson, LL. D. (London), Solicitor and Clerk to the Shoreditch *Medical Publications of The F. A. Davit Co., Philadelphia.*

Sanitary Authority; Law Examiner for the British Institute of Public Health, etc.; ami Cecil H. Cribb, B.sc. (London), F.I.C., F.C.S., Public Analyst to the Strand District, etc. Crown Octavo. About 300 pages.

Price, in United States and Canada, HI.00, net; Great Britain, 8s.; France, » fr. 50.

ROHE—Text-Book of Hygiene.

A Comprehensive Treatise on the Principles and Practice of Preventive Medicine from an American Stand point. By George H. Roue, M.D., Professor of Obstetrics and Hygiene in the College of Physicians and Surgeons, Baltimore; Member of the American Public Health Association, etc. Third Edition, carefully revised and enlarged, with many Illustrations and valuable Tables. Royal Octavo. Over 450 pages. Extra Cloth.

Price, in United States and Canada, S3.00, net; Great Britain, 14s.; France, 18 fr. 60.

ROHE—A Practical flanual of Diseases of the Skin.

By George II. Roue, M.D., assisted by J. Williams Lord, A.B., M.D., Lecturer on Dermatology and Bandaging in the College of Physicians and Surgeons, Baltimore, etc. 12mo. Over 300 pages. Extra Cloth.

Price, in United States and Canada, »1.»5, net; Great Britain, 6s. 6d.; France, *l* fr. »5.

SAJOUS—Hay Fever and its Successful Treatment,

By Superficial Organic Alteration Of The Nasal Mucous MemBrane. By Charles E. Sajous, M.D., Chief Editor "Annual of the Universal Medical Sciences"; formerly Lecturer on Rhinology and Laryngology in the Jefferson Medical College, etc. With 13 Engravings on Wood. 12mo. Extra Cloth. Price, in United States and Canada, m. 00, net; Great Britain, 6.; France, 6 fr. 20.

SCHUSTER—When is marriage Permissible after Syphilis?

By Dr. Schuster, of Aix-la-Chapelle. Translated from the German by C. Renner, M.D., London. 8vo. 32 pages. Price, 25 cents net, or 1 shilling.

SENN—Principles of Surgery.

By N. Senn, M.D., Ph.D., Professor of

Principles of Surgery and Surgical Pathology in Rush Medical College, Chicago, Ill.; Professor of Surgery in the Chicago Polyclinic, etc. Royal Octavo. With 109 line Wood-Engravings. 624 pages. Price, in United States and Canada, Cloth, 94.50, net; Sheep or HalfRussia, W5.50, net. Great Britain, Cloth, 24s. 6d.; Sheep or HalfRussia, 30s. France, Cloth, 27 fr. 20; Sheep or Half-Russia, 33 fr. 10.

SENN—Tuberculosis of the Bones and Joints.

By N. Senn, M.D., Ph.D., author of a text-book on the "Principles of Surgery," etc. Royal Octavo. Over 500 pages. Illustrated with 107 Engravings, many of them colored.

Price, in United States and Canada, Extra Cloth, S4.00, net; Sheep or Half-Russia, S5.00, net. Great Britain, Cloth, 22s. 6d.; Sheep or Half-Russia, 28s. France, Cloth, 24 ft. 60; Sheep or Half-Russia, 30 fr. 30.

Medical Publications of The F. A. Davis Co., Philadelphia. SHOEMAKER—Heredity, Health, and Personal Beauty.

Including the Selection of the Best Cosmetics for the Skin, Hair, Moils, and All Parts Relating to the Body. By John V. Shoemaker, A.M., M.D., Professor of Materia Medica, Pharmacology, Therapeutics, and Clinical Medicine, and Clinical Professor of Diseases of the Skin in the Medico-Chirurgical College of Philadelphia, etc. Royal Octavo. 425 pages.

Price, in United States and Canada, Cloth, S2.50, net; Half-Morocco, S3.50, net. Great Britain, Cloth, 14s.; Half-Morocco, 19s. 6d. France, Cloth, 15 fr.; Half-Morocco, 22 fr.

SHOEMAKER—Ointments and Oleates,

Especially in Diseases of the Skin. By John V. Shoemaker, A.M., M.D. Second Edition, revised and enlarged. 298 pages. 12mo. Extra Cloth.

Price, in United States and Canada, S1.150, net; Great Britain, 8s. 6d.; France, 9 fr. 35.

SHOEMAKER—Hateria Hedica and Therapeutics.

With Especial Reference to the Clinical Application of Drugs. By John V. Shoemaker, A.M., M.D., Professor of Materia Medica, Pharmacology and Therapeutics, and Clinical Medicine, and Clinical Professor of Diseases of the Skin in the Medico-Chirurgical College of Philadelphia, etc. Second Edition, Thoroughly Revised. In Two Volumes. Royal Octavo. Nearly 1100 pages. The volumes may be purchased separately.

Volume 1 (354 pages) is devoted to Pharmacy, general Pharmacology and Therapeutics, and remedial agents not properly classed with drugs.

Price, in United States and Canada, Extra Cloth, V2.50, net; Sheep, S3.25, net. Great Britain, Extra Cloth, 14s.; Sheep, 18s. France, Extra Cloth, 16 fr. 20; Sheep, 20 fr. 20.

Volume II (700 pages) is wholly taken up with the consideration of drugs, each remedy being studied from three points of view,—viz., the Preparations, or Materia Medica; the Physiology and Toxicology, or Pharmacology; and, lastly, its Therapy.

Price, in United States and Canada, Extra Cloth, S3.50, net; Sheep, S4.50, not. Great Britain, Extra Cloth, 19s.; Sheep, 25s. France, Extra Cloth, 22 fr. 40; Sheep, 28 fr. 60. Each volume is thoroughly and carefully indexed with clinical and general indexes, and the second volume contains a most valuable and exhaustive table of doses extending over several double-column octavo pages.

SNITH—Physiology of the Domestic Animals.

A Text-Book for Veterinary and Medical Students and Practitioners. By Robert Meade Smith, A.M., M.D., formerly Professor of Comparative Physiology in University of Pennsylvania, etc. Royal Octavo. Over 950 pages. Profusely illustrated with more than 400 fine Wood-Engravings, some of them Colored. Price, in United States and Canada, Cloth, S5.00, not; Sheep, S6.00, net. Great Britain, Cloth, 28s.; Sheep, 32s. France, Cloth, 30 fr. 30; Sheep, 36 fr. 20.

SOZINSKEY—fledical Symbolism.

Historical Studies in the Arts of Healing and Hygiene. By Thomas S. SozinsKey, M.D., Ph.D., Author of "The Culture of Beauty," "The Care and Culture of *Medical Publications of The F. A. Davit Co.. Philadelphia.*

Children," etc. 12mo. Nearly 200 pages. Extra Cloth. Appropriately illustrated with thirty (30) new Wood-Engravings.

Price, in United States and Canada, 1. 00, net; Great Britain, 6s.; France, 6 fr. 20.

STEWART—Obstetric Synopsis.

A Complete Conipend. By John 8. Stewart, M.D., late Demonstrator of Obstetrics in the Medico-Chirurgical College of Philadelphia; with an introductory note by William S. Stewart, A. M., M.D., Emeritus Professor of Obstetrics and Gynaecology in the Medico-Chirurgical College of Philadelphia. 42 Illustrations. 202 pages. 12mo. Extra Blue Cloth.

Price, in United States and Canada, S1.00, net; Great Britain, 6s. France, 6 fr. 20.

STRAUB—Symptom Register and Case Record.

Designed by D. W. Straub, M.D. Giving in plain view, on one side of the sheet x 10% inches, the Clinical Record of the sick, including Date, Name, Residence, Occupation, Symptoms, Inspection (Auscultation and Percussion), History, Respiration, Pulse, Temperature, Diagnosis, Prognosis, Treatment (special and general), and Remarks, all conveniently arranged, and with ample room for recording, at each call, for four different calls, each item named above, the whole forming a clinical history of individual cases of great value to every Practitioner.

Published in stiff Board Tablets, of 50 sheets each, at 50 cents, net, per tablet; and in Book-form, flexible binding, with Alphabetical Marginal Index, at 75 cents, net.

THRESH—Water Supplies.

By J. C. Thresh, D.Sc.Lond., M.B. . F.I.C., F.C.S., Lecturer in Sanitary Science, King's College, London, etc. City Authorities, Town Councils, Levy Courts, County Councils, Farmers, Owners of Villas or Private Residences in the Country, Settlers in newly-opened Districts, Colonists, etc., will find this little book of extreme value, as it contains practical hints with excellent illustrations by the score. Illustrated. One Volume. Crown Octavo. About 300 pages. Cloth.

Price, in the United States and Canada, W2.00, net; Great Britain, 8s.; France, 9 fr. 50.

Transactions of the neetings of the British Laryngological Association.

Volume I. 1891. Royal 8vo. 108 pages. Cloth. Price, 2s. 6d. (75 cents, net).
Volume II, 1892. Royal 8vo. 100 pages. Cloth. Price, 2s. 6d. (75 cents, net).
Volume III, 1893. Royal 8vo. 106 pages. Price, 2s. 6d. (75 cents, net).
The three volumes together, 6s. (S2.00, net).

ULTZHANN—The Neuroses of the denito-Urinary System in the Hale.

With Sterility and Impotence. By Dr. Ultzmann, Professor of Genitourinary Diseases in the University of Vienna. Translated, with tho author's permission, by Gardner W. Allen, M.D., Surgeon in the Genito-Urinary Department, Boston Dispensary. Dlustrated. 12mo. Extra Cloth.

Price, In United States and Canada. S1.00, net; Great Britain, 6s.; France, 6 fr. 20.
(U)

Hedical Publications of the F. A. Davis Co., Philadelphia. VOUGHT—Chapter on Cholera for Lay Readers.

History, Symptoms, Prevention, and Treatment of the Disease. By Waltib Vought, Ph.B., M.D., late Medical Director and Physician-m-Chargc of the Fire Island Quarantine Station, Port of New York; Fellow of the New York Academy of Medicine, etc. Illustrated. 12mo. 106 pages. Flexible Cloth.

Price, in United States and Canada, 75 cents, net; Great Britain, 4s.; France, 5 fr.

WITHERSTINE-International Pocket Medical Formulary.

Arranged Therapeutically. By C. Sumner Witherstine, A.M., M.D., Visiting Physician of the Home for the Aged, Qermantown, Philadelphia; late House Surgeon to Charity Hospital, New York, etc. Including more than 1800 formulas from several hundred well-known authorities. With an Appendix containing a Posological Table, the newer remedies included; Formulae and Doses of Hypodermatic Medication, including the newer remedies; Uses of the Hypodermatic Syringe, etc. 275 printed pages, besides extra blank leaves for new formulas. Elegantly printed, with red lines, edges, and borders. Illustrated. Bound in Leather, with Side-Flap.

Price, in United States and Canada, S2.00, net; Great Britain, 1is. Cd.; France, 12 fr. 40.

YOUNG—Synopsis of Human Anatomy. liei ng a Complete Compend of Anatomy, including the Anatomy of the Viscera, and Numerous Tables. By James K. Young, M.D., Instructor in Orthopaedic Surgery and Assistant Demonstrator of Surgery, University of Pennsylvania, etc. Illustrated with 76 Wood-Engravings. 320 pages. 12mo. Extra Cloth.

Price, in United States and Canada, S1.40, net; Great Britain. 8s. 6d.; France, » fr. 25.

The following Publications are Sold Only by Subscription, or Sent Direct on Receipt of Price, Shipping Expenses Prepaid.

Annual of the Universal Medical Sciences.

A Yearly Report of the Progress of the General Sanitary Sciences Throughout the World. Edited by Charles E. Sajous, M.D., formerly lecturer on Laryngology and Rhinology in Jefferson Medical College, Philadelphia, etc., and Seventy Associate Editors, assisted by over Two Hundred Corresponding Editore and Collaborators. In Five Royal Octavo Volumes of about 500 pages each. Illustrated with Chromo-Lithographs, Engravings. Maps, Charts, and Diagrams. Being intended to enable any physician to possess, at a moderate cost, a complete Contemporary History of Universal Medicine.

Subscription Price per year (including the " Universal Medical Journal" for one year), in United States, Cloth, 5 vols., Royal Octavo, S15.00; Half-Russia, *910.00.* Canada (duty paid), Cloth, S16.00; HalfRussia, S21.00. Great Britain, Cloth, £4 7s.; Half-Russia, 5 15s. France, Cloth, 93 fr. 95; Half-Russia, 124 fr. 35. The "Universal Medical Journal" is a Monthly Review of the practical branches of Medicine and Surgery, and is supplied free to the subscribers to the "Annual"; to non-subscribers, S2.00 per year; Great Britain, 8s. 6d.

Medical Publications of The F. A. Davis Co., Philadelphia. ADAMS—History of the Life of D. Hayes Agnew, n.D., LL. D.

By J. Howe Adahs, M.D. A fascinating life-history of one of the world's greatest surgeons. Royal Octavo. 376 pages. Handsomely printed, with Portraits and other Illustrations.

Price, in United States and Canada, Extra Cloth, S2.80, net.; Half-Morocco, Gilt Top, S3.50.net. Great Britain, Cloth, 14s.; Half-Morocco, 19s. 6d. France, Cloth, 15 fr.; Half-Morocco, 82 fr.

KRAFFT-EBINQ—Psychopathia Sexualis.

With Especial Reference to Contrary Sexual Instinct: A Medico-Legal Study of Sexual Insanity. By Dr. R. Von Krafft-ebing, Professor of Psychiatry and Neurology, University of Vienna. Authorized Translation of the Seventh Enlarged and Revised German Edition, by Charlks Gilbert Ciiaddock, M.D., Professor of Norvous and Mental Diseases, Marion-Sima College of Medicine, St. Louis. One Royal Octavo Volume. 432 pages.

Price, in the United States and Canada, Cloth, S3.00, net; Sheep, S4.00, net. Great Britain, Cloth, 17s.; Sheep, 2Is. France, Cloth,18fr.60; Sheep, 24 fr. 60.

RANNEY—Lectures on Nervous Diseases.

From the Stand-Point of Cerebral and Spinal Localization, and the Later Methods Employed in the Diagnosis and Treatment of these Affections. By AmBrose L. Ranney, A.M., M.D., formerly Professor of the Anatomy and Physiology of the Nervous System in the New York Post-Graduate Medical

School and Hospital, etc.; Author of "The Applied Anatomy of the Nervous System," "Practical Medical Anatomy," etc. Profusely Illustrated with Original Diagrams and Sketches in Color by the author, carefully selected Wood-Engravings, and Reproduced Photographs of Typical Cases. Royal Octavo. 780 pages.

Price, in United States and Canada, Cloth, S5.50; Sheep, S8.50; Half-Russia, S7.00. Great Britain, Cloth. 32s. ; Sheep, 38s.; Half-Russia, 40s. France, Cloth, 34 fr. 70; Sheep. 40 fr. 45; Half-Russia, 43 fr. 30.

SAJOUS—Lectures on the Diseases of the Nose and Throat.

Delivered at the Jefferson Medical College, Philadelphia. By Charles E. SAJOUS, M.D., formerly Lecturer on Rhinology and Laryngology in Jefferson Medical College; Vice-President of the American Laryngological Association, etc. Illustrated with 100 Chnnno-Lithographs, from Oil-Paintiugs by the author, and 93 Engravings on Wood. One handsome Royal Octavo volume.

Price, in United States and Canada, Cloth, S4.00; Half-Russia, S5.00. Great Britain, Cloth, 22s. 6d.; Sheep or Half-Russia, 28s. France, Cloth, 24 fr. 60; Half-Russia, 30 fr. 30.

SCHRENCK-NOTZING— Suggestive Therapeutics in Psychopathia Sexualis.

By Dr. A. Von Schrenck-notzing, of Munich. Authorized Translation of the List Enlarged and Revised German Edition, by Charles Gilbert Chaddock, M. D., Professor of Nervous and Mental Diseases, Marion-Sims College of Medicine, St. Louia, etc. An invaluable supplementary volume to Dr. R. Von KrafftEbing's masterly treatise on "Psychopathia Sexualis" (also translated by Dr. Chaddock). A kind of hand-book of the treatment of Sexual Pathology upon sound and effective principles. Royal Octavo. About 350 pages. Nearly Ready. *Medical Publications of The F. A. Davis Co., Philadelphia.* STANTON—Practical and Scientific Physiognomy.

Or, How to lie ad Faces. By Mary Olmsted Stanton. Copiously Illustrated. Two large Royal Octavo volumes, l:£ii pages. To physicians the diagnostic information conveyed in these volumes is invaluable. To the general reader each page opens a new train of ideas. (This book has no reference whatever to Phrenology.)

Price, in United States and Canada, Cloth, S9.00; Sheep, »11.00; Half. Russia, S13.00. (ircat Britain, Clotb, 48s.: Sheep, 58s.; Half-Russia, 63s. Franco, Cloth, 30 tr. 30; Sheep, 3(1 fr. 40; Half-Russia, 43 fr. 30.

Journal of Laryngology, Rhinology, and Otology.

An Analytical Record of Current Literature Relating to the Throat, Nose, and Ear. Issued on the First of Each Month. Edited by Dr. Norris Wolfenden, of ljondou, and Dr. John Macintyre, of Glasgow, with the active aid and cooperation of Drs. Dundas Grant, Barclay J. Baron, and Hunter Mackenzie.

Price, 13s. or S3.00 per annum (inclusive of postage). For single copies, however, a charge of Is. 3d. (30 cents) will be made. Sample Copy, 25 cents.

The Medical Bulletin.

A Monthly Journal of Medicine and Surgery. Edited by John V. Shoemaker, A.M., M.D. Articles by the best practical writers procurable. Every article as brief as Is consistent with the preservation of its scientific value. Therapeutic notes by the leaders of the medical profession throughout tko world. These and many other unique features help to keep THE Medical Bulletin in its present position as the leading Medical Monthly of the world. Subscribe now.

Terms, S1.00 a Year in advance, in United States, Canada, and Mexico; England and Australia, 5 shillings; France, 6 francs; Japan, 1 yen; Germany, 5 marks; Holland, 3 ilorins.

The Universal Medical Journal.

A Monthly Magazine of the Progress of Every Branch of Medicine in all Parts of tho World. Edited by Charles K Sajous, M.D., Edltor-in-Chief of the "Annual of the Universal Medical Sciences. "

Subscription Price, in United States, S2.00 per year; in other countries of the Postal Union, 8s. 6d. or 10 fr. 50.

Medical Times and Hospital Gazette.

The Journal of tho Medical Practitioners' Association. Published Weekly at 11 Adam Street, Strand, London, W. C.

Price, 2d.; by post, 2yjd. Per annum, post-free, 8s.; half-yearty, 4s. 6d.; quarterly, 2s. 6d. Abroad, 12s. 6d. per annum (W3.00).

Lightning Source UK Ltd.
Milton Keynes UK
UKOW02f2357100214

226247UK00007B/556/P